Eldercare Technology for Clinical Practitioners

AGING MEDICINE

Robert Pignolo, MD, PhD; Mary Ann Forciea, MD; Jerry C. Johnson, MD,
Series Editors

Majd Alwan · Robin A. Felder
Editors

Eldercare Technology for Clinical Practitioners

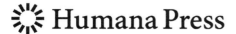 Humana Press

Editors

Majd Alwan
Center for Aging Services
  Technologies (CAST)
Washington, DC

Robin A. Felder
Department of Pathology
University of Virgina Health
  Sciences Center
Charlottesville, VA

Series Editors

Robert J. Pignolo, MD, PhD
Assistant Professor of Medicine
Department of Medicine
Division of Geriatric Medicine
University of Pennsylvania Health System

Jerry C. Johnson, MD
Professor of Medicine
Chief, Division of Geriatric Medicine
Senior Fellow, Institute on Aging
University of Pennsylvania Health System

Mary Ann Forciea, MD
Clinical Associate Professor of Medicine
Division of Geriatric Medicine
University of Pennsylvania Health System

ISBN: 978-1-58829-898-0   e-ISBN: 978-1-59745-233-5

Library of Congress Control Number: 2007940426

Preface

Background: The majority of our increasing elder adult population requires some degree of formal and/or informal care because of loss of function as a result of failing health. According to the Centers for Disease Control (CDC), nearly three-quarters of elder adults suffer from one or more chronic diseases. Examples include arthritis, hypertension, and diabetes, to name a few. The cost and burden of caring for elder adults is steadily increasing.

Changes in the Medicare system led to a shift in the responsibility for care from institutions (nursing homes, etc.) to the community (individuals and families). The role of informal caregivers in providing care to the elder adult population has greatly increased in the past two decades. Consequently, informal caregivers have come to be viewed as an unpaid extension of professional caregivers, providing most of the care to elder adults requiring long-term care. In fact, national databases derived from different sources have provided unequivocal evidence that family and friends are the sole care providers for about three-quarters of all community-dwelling elder adults. Informal caregivers have experienced increased physical burdens and emotional strains because of this shift in long-term elder care responsibilities. Furthermore, healthcare providers are faced with a shrinking professional caregiving work force at the same time.

On the contrary, the proportion of the world's population of individuals over the age of 60 years is expected to double by 2030 to 20%. In the USA, the number of elder adults is expected to grow to 108 million over the next 15 years, which represents 45% of the adult population. Elder adults currently account for 60% of the overall healthcare spending in the USA. Appropriate management of chronic disease in older adults can reduce the US health care bill by up to 50%. Furthermore, 92% of these elder adults live alone in their own apartments, homes, independent living facilities, or assisted living facilities, including about 50% of those 75 years and older. Such statistics demonstrate an urgent need for innovative telehealth/telecare tools that enable elder adults to live independently and maximize caregivers' efficacy by providing timely health information and delivering more effective care. This change in the demographics and its potential economic impact on industrialized nations has prompted active research in automated systems for functional and health status monitoring and assistance, enabled by recent technological advancement.

In the meantime, advances in sensor, communication, and information technologies have created opportunities to develop novel tools enabling remote management and monitoring of chronic diseases, emergency conditions, and the delivery of health care. In-home health assessment and monitoring has the added benefit of measuring individualized health status and reporting it to the primary care provider and caregivers alike, allowing timelier and targeted preventive interventions. Health monitoring in home environments can be accomplished by a) ambulatory monitors that utilize wearable sensors and devices to record physiological signals; b) sensors embedded in the home environment and furnishings to unobtrusively collect behavioral and physiological data; or c) a combination of the two.

Aim and scope: This book addresses technologies targeted at the assessment, early detection, and the mitigation of common geriatric conditions including decline in functional abilities, gait, mobility, sleep disturbance, vision impairment, hearing loss, falls, and cognitive decline. This book not only describes the state of both embedded and wearable technologies, including technologies under research and on the brink of translation into products, but also focuses on research showing the potential utility of these technologies in the field.

Chapter 1 presents an introduction and reviews the statistics that make a compelling case for development and utilization of technologies for the geriatric care. Chapter 2 presents a comprehensive review of functional assessment instruments and promising technologies used in functional assessment of elders. Chapter 3 covers mobility and gait assessment technologies, whereas Chapter 4 reviews mobility aid technologies for the elderly. In Chapter 5, we review sleep disorders in older age and sleep assessment technologies, with emphasis on in-home assessment technologies. Chapter 6 presents a comprehensive review of age-related changes in vision and corrective technologies, whereas Chapter 7 addresses the management of hearing loss in older age. Chapter 8 is dedicated to falls, fall detection, and fall prevention technologies. Finally, Chapter 9 addresses emerging computer-based cognitive assessment technologies.

We believe, and hope, that this work will fill a gap in the knowledge and will be invaluable to Eldercare practitioners, as well as medical student studying Geriatrics and interested in gerotechnology, social studies, students studying gerontology and interested in gerontechnology, and nursing students interested in Geriatric Nursing, in addition to engineering students interested in Eldercare Technologies, and researchers from a broad spectrum of disciplines, particularly those interested in field experience and the end-user's perspective. This volume comes at a time when interest in Eldercare Technology and the need for effective and appropriate technologies especially are peaking.

Washington, District of Columbia   Majd Alwan
Charlottesville, Virginia   Robin A. Felder

Contents

Contributors

Vered Aharonson, Ph.D., Department of Software Engineering, Tel Aviv Academic College of Engineering, Afeka, Israel

Gregory L. Alexander, Ph.D., R.N., Assistant Professor, Sinclair School of Nursing, Columbia, MO

Majd Alwan, Ph.D., Director, Center for Aging Services Technologies (CAST), Washington, DC

Matthew H. Bakke, Ph.D., Associate Professor, Gallaudet University, Department of Hearing, Speech and Language Sciences, Director, Rehabilitation Engineering Research Center (RERC) on Hearing Enhancement, Washington, DC

Scott J. Bally, Ph.D., Associate Professor, Gallaudet University, Department of Hearing, Speech and Language Sciences, Washington, DC

Claire M. Bernstein, Ph.D., Research Audiologist, Gallaudet University, Department of Hearing, Speech and Language Sciences, Washington, DC

Marybeth Brown, Ph.D., Professor, Physical Therapy, School of Health Professions, Columbia, MO

Kathryn Burks, R.N., Ph.D., School of Nursing, University of Missouri, Columbia, MO

Amy Corcoran, M.D., Geriatric Fellow, Department of Medicine, Division of Geriatrics, University of Pennsylvania, Philadelphia, PA

George Demiris, Ph.D., Associate Professor, Biobehavioral Nursing and Health Systems, School of Nursing & Biomedical and Health Informatics, School of Medicine, University of Washington, Seattle, WA

Marc Hamilton, Ph.D., Associate Professor, Biomedical Sciences, Dalton Cardiovascular Research Investigator & College of Veterinary Medicine, University of Missouri, Columbia, MO

Zhihai He, Ph.D., Assistant Professor, Department of Electrical and Computer Engineering, University of Missouri, Columbia, MO

Brian K. Hensel, Ph.D., M.S.P.H., Post-Doctoral Fellow in Health Informatics, University of Missouri-Columbia, Columbia, MO

Cunjun Huang, Ph.D., Department of Mechanical and Aerospace Engineering, University of Virginia, Charlottesville, VA

D. Casey Kerrigan, M.D., M.S., University of Virginia, School of Medicine, Department of Physical Medicine and Rehabilitation, Charlottesville, VA

Bruce Kinosian, M.D., Associate Professor, Divisions of General Internal Medicine and Geriatrics, University of Pennsylvania, School of Medicine, Philadelphia, PA

Steven M. Koenig, M.D., FCCP, Professor of Internal Medicine, University of Virginia Health System, The Department of Internal Medicine, Division of Pulmonary & Critical Care, Charlottesville, VA

Amos D. Korczyn, M.D., B.Sc., Professor, Sieratzki Chair of Neurology, Tel-Aviv University Medical School, Ramat-Aviv, Israel

Jia Lee, Ph.D., R.N., Assistant Professor, Sinclair School of Nursing, Columbia, MO

Richard Lindsay, M.D., Former Chair of Geriatric Medicine, School of Medicine, University of Virginia, Charlottesville, VA

David Mack, M.S., Ph.D., Graduate Research Assistant, Medical Automation Research Center, University of Verginia, Charlottesville, VA

Kate W. Paylo, D.O., University of Virginia, School of Medicine, Department of Physical Medicine and Rehabilitation, Charlottesville, VA

Janet L. Pray, Ph.D., Professor, Gallaudet University, Department of Social Work, Washington, DC

Prabhu Rajendran, M.S., Graduate Research Assistant, Medical Automation Research Center, University of Virginia, Charlottesville, VA

Marilyn Rantz, R.N., Ph.D., F.A.A.N., Professor, Sinclair School of Nursing and Family and Community Medicine, S 406 Sinclair School of Nursing, University of Missouri-Columbia, Columbia, MO

Patrick O. Riley, Ph.D., Research Associate Professor, University of Virginia, School of Medicine, Department of Physical Medicine and Rehabilitation, Charlottesville, VA

Pradip Sheth, Ph.D., Department of Mechanical and Aerospace Engineering, University of Virginia, Charlottesville, VA

Marjorie Skubic, Ph.D., Associate Professor, Electrical and Computer Engineering Department, Columbia, MO

Harry W. Tyrer, Ph.D., Professor, Department of Electrical and Computer Engineering, University of Missouri, Columbia, MO

Glenn Wasson, Ph.D., Department of Computer Science, University of Virginia, Charlottesville, VA

Stanley Woo, Ph.D., Clinical Associate Professor, Chief, Low Vision Rehabilitation Services, Director, Center for Sight Enhancement, University of Houston College of Optometry, Houston, TX

Jie Yu, B.S.N., R.N., Doctoral Student, Sinclair School of Nursing, Columbia, MO

List of Acronyms and Abbreviations

AASM	American Academy of Sleep Medicine
ABR	Auditory brainstem response
AD	Alzheimer's disease
ADLs	Activities of daily living
AGC	Automatic gain control
AI	Apnea index
ALD	Assistive listening devices
ALS	Assistive listening systems
AMD	Age-related macular degeneration
ARES	Apnea Risk Evaluation System
ASDA	American Sleep Disorders Association
AVC	Automatic volume control
BCG	Ballistocardiogram
BPPV	Benign paroxysmal positional vertigo
BOS	Bed Occupancy Sensors
BTE	Behind-the-ear
BTS	Bioptic telescopic spectacle
CBS	Charles Bonnet Syndrome
CCTV	Closed circuit televisions
CDC	Centers for Disease Control
CES-D	Center for Epidemiologic Studies Depression
CIC	Completely-in-the-canal
CLVT	Certified low vision therapist
CNA	Certified nursing assistant
CPAP	Constant Positive Airway Pressure
CRT	Cathode ray tube
CSF	Contrast sensitivity function
CSOA	Communication Self-Assessment Scales for Older Adults
DAQ	Data acquisition
DYS	Familial Torsion Dystonia
ECG	Electrocardiogram
EDS	excessive daytime sleepiness
EEG	Electroencephalogram
EGM	Electromyography

EMG	Electromyogram
ENG	Electronystagmography
ETDRS	Early Treatment of Diabetic Retinopathy Study
EV	Eccentric viewing
FDA	Food and Drug Administration
FEM	Finite element model
FFT	Fast Fourier transform
FM	Frequency modulated radio frequencies
FRA	Fall Risk Assessment
FRT	Functional Reach Test
FSQ	Functional Status Questionnaire
GRF	Ground reaction force
HAT	Hearing Assistance Technology
HATNAP	Hearing Assistive Technology Needs Assessment Profile
HF	High frequency
HI	Hypopnea index
HLAA	Hearing Loss Association of America
HRVI	Heart rate variation index
IADL	Instrumental activities of daily living
IL	Induction loops
ILSA	Independent Lifestyle Assistant
IR	Infrared light
ISI	Intermittent snoring index
IT	Information technology
ITC	In-the-canal
ITE	In-the-ear
JND	Just-noticeable difference
LED	Light emitting diodes
LPL	Lipoprotein lipase
LVR	Low vision rehabilitation
MARC	Medical Automation Research Center
MCI	Mild cognitive impairment
MET	Metabolic Equivalent Test
MMSE	Mini-Mental State Examination
MSLT	Multiple sleep latency test
MU	University of Missouri
NAPS	Non-invasive Analysis of Physiological Signals
NIH	National Institutes of Health
NEPA	Non-exercise physical activity
NSF	National Sleep Foundation
OAE	Otoacoustic emissions testing
OSAHS	Obstructive sleep apnea-hypopnea syndrome
OSA	Obstructive sleep apnea
ODI	Oxygen desaturation index
PAPAW	Push-rim activated power assist wheelchair

PFQ	Physical Functioning Questionnaire
PLMS	
PPT	Physical Performance Test
PM	POLY-MESAM
PSG	Polysomnography
RERA	Respiratory effort-related arousal
ROC	Right outer canthus
REM	Rapid eye movement
RSVP	Rapid serial visual presentation
SCSB	Static Charge Sensitive Bed
SDB	Sleep disordered breathing
SHHS	Sleep Health Heart Study
SIMBAD	Smart Inactivity Monitor Using Array Based Detectors
SL	Sleep latency
SPMSQ	Short Portable Mental Status Questionnaire
SPPB	Short Physical Performance Battery test
TIB	Time in bed
TMJ	Temporomandibular joint
TRT	Tinnitus retraining therapy
TST	Total sleep time
TUG	Timed Up and Go
UARS	Upper airway resistance syndrome
ULF	Ultra Low Frequency
VMS	Video magnifier systems
WOMAC	Western Ontario and McMaster Universities Osteoarthritis Index

Chapter 1
Introduction

Richard Lindsay

Increases in the number and proportion of our population over age 65, and the dynamic changes within the aging population itself represent the most dramatic change in American society in this century. And projections call for additional dramatic graying of American well into the twenty-first century.

John W. Rowe, MD

"I want to live at home!" This phrase is uttered over and over again by senior citizens, and is their preference. I am hopeful that it will become the preference of more healthcare professionals, insurers, and those who make policy. The concept of aging-in-place has been defined as "living where you have lived for many years, or living in a non-healthcare environment, using products, services and conveniences to allow or enable the elderly to not have to move as circumstances change" [1]. New smart home technology exists in the form of emergency assistance notification, medication reminders, fall prevention, and detection. The technology allows for continuous monitoring of patients and for greatly improved psychosocial interaction. With this as a background, my introduction will review some of the factors impacting "aging in place" and thus will indicate the importance of the author's detailed review of the role that technology can play in helping us reach our goals of better health care for the elderly and aging in place.

It is evident that there is an Aging Tsunami underway and it is very close to reaching the harbor where tsunamis cause the greatest amount of damage. The challenge for our society will be how we prepare for, and meet, this aging wave and its accompanying age-prevalent problems. Will the U.S. be able to perfect a system of health care that is truly affordable, responsive, caring, and available for our population and particularly the elderly?

In 1910, the average live expectancy for woman was 47 years of age and today it is close to 80 years; for men the average is 72 years. In 1900, there were 3 million elderly or one in every 25 Americans. The number had increased, by 1994, to 33.2 million or 1 in 8. By 2030, 1 in 5 Americans will be over 65 years. Predictions,

Richard Lindsay
Former Chair of Geriatric Medicine, School of Medicine, University of Virginia, Charlottesville, VA
e-mail: rwl3w@virginia.edu

From: *Aging Medicine, Eldercare Technology for Clinical Practitioners,*
Edited by: M. Alwan and R. Felder © Humana Press, Totowa, NJ

from demographers, indicate that by the year 2050 the elderly will number some 80 million.

The most rapidly growing segment in the U.S. population is those 85 years and older, which grew 274% from the years 1960 to 1994. This group has been called the "old old" and numbered some 3 million in 1994. It is predicted to number 19 million by the year 2050, including survivors of the "baby boom." These baby boomers are the birth cohort born between 1946 and 1964 who gave a tsunami-like picture to the aging U.S. population. The first of the baby boomers will turn 65 years old in 2011, and people aged 65 and over are projected to represent 20% of the total U.S. population in 2030 compared with 12% in 2003. This sudden dramatic increase in our elderly population has called into question the solvency of the major entitlement programs: Medicare, Medicaid, and Social Security. This will stress the ability of our health care system to provide quality services.

This "old old" subset of the population is also the one that often demands the greatest outlay of health care resources because they are often the ones with the greatest functional impairment and in need of the largest support network. This functional impairment is largely due to an increase in chronic disease. About 80% of seniors have at least one chronic health condition, and 59% have at least two chronic health conditions which often lead to disability. Conditions including arthritis, hypertension, heart disease, diabetes, and respiratory disorders represent the new focus on medicine; the care and management of chronic illness which frequently takes place outside of hospitals. Chronic illnesses lend themselves to monitoring by the patient and/or their caregiver and other members of the health care team. This offers new and exciting opportunities to apply technology as you will see as you read this book.

There is one other important aspect of the aging tsunami that deserves comment: the fact that the next generation of elderly will be much more heterogeneous than the last. There will be an explosive growth in the population of minority elderly. The white elderly will double between 1990 and 2050 and the numbers of African-Americans will triple. The numbers of older Hispanics and Asians will increase by a factor of five. This will need to be taken into account when designing programs and health care materials, training personnel, and placing instruction on equipment if the health care to these populations is to be successful.

The absolute numbers of elderly who will be in need of services and care brings me to the other critical point in this introduction. A recent International Commission on Global Aging declared, "The major social crisis of the twenty-first century will be the by-product of labor shortages" [2]. Unless there are adequate numbers of individuals trained in the proper care of geriatric patients, the whole system will be in danger. There are approximately 7,600 certified geriatricians in the U.S. today. Estimates put the need for geriatricians in the year 2030 at approximately 36,000. The total number of individuals in geriatric fellowship training programs in the U.S. was 334 in 2005.

The situation is similar in nursing, with a current dramatic shortage of RNs and a prediction of an additional shortage of between 800,000 and 1 million registered nurses by 2020. The current nursing force is aging and many plan to retire within 10 years. Other professional careers that play a key role in caring for the elderly, including pharmacy, dentistry, chiropractic, podiatry, optometry, nutrition, and occupational and speech therapy all could face potential personnel shortages or could benefit from additional geriatric educational content in their training programs. These disciplines are vital members of the health care team for the elderly and these shortages could further compromise the maintenance of function and health for our aging population.

The same problems face us in the supply and retention of Certified Nursing Assistants (CNAs) who give the vast majority of hands on care in nursing homes. At a time when Americans want to age-in-place and be cared for at home, the agencies that provide this care are closing or struggling because of a shortage of home health aides. Given the long training periods involved in some of these career paths and the low wage scale in others and being aware of the already existent shortages of those caregivers who directly provide the hands on care only serves to emphasize the crisis nature of the situation. Solutions include attention to additional geriatric content as a requirement for certification and licensure and earlier exposure of high school students to the rewards of a career in the many fields discussed above. We must also address the economic issues of wages and benefits. Until we solve the personnel problem, other discussions about care for the elderly will represent a classic case of the "cart before the horse" and new programs to care for the elderly will be destined to failure.

Future planning must also consider developing different ways of providing care in different settings. The role of technology in offsetting personnel shortages, linking the home and the health care system, providing continuing education to patients and caregivers, decreasing transportation usage, and monitoring chronic illness will need funding and further research. The goal is better care and cost saving.

Today, we are in the space age of technology for the care of the elderly. We have moved beyond the sphygmomanometer, oral thermometer, wheel chairs, and walkers. New developments in sensors that allow following patient's gait motion, sleep, vital signs, and location can and will provide new means of monitoring and connecting the patient with their health care system. The internet and electronic systems that facilitate information exchange for the elderly patient or their caregiver are only beginning to be utilized and offer great potential. New assistive devices can help clean a house, enhance personal safety, and aid in medication compliance. These represent just a few of the ways technology will meet the demand of "I want to stay at home".

There are many challenges that have and will delay technology's role in the care of the elderly; including reimbursement for using technology, the development of user-friendly devices and keeping the technology affordable. Fortunately, the baby boomers have grown up with technology and use it in many aspects of their daily lives, and this will facilitate its employment.

Technology is and will be a major partner in the care of the elderly and our health care system in the future. The challenges will be in providing adequate resources for continuing research into its application in the care of the elderly and developing strong working relationships between the health care system and the researchers. The authors' contributions contained in this volume represent significant steps toward meeting these challenges.

References

1. Aging in place. Available at: http://www.semiorresource.com/agingimpl.htm. Accessed August 21, 2006.
2. Mondale W, Hashimoto R, Pohl KO. Summary Report of the co-chairmen and findings and recommendations of the CSIS Commission on Global Aging. Washington DC: Global Aging Initiative Center for Strategic and International Studies; August 29, 2001.

Chapter 2
Functional Assessment Technologies

Marilyn Rantz, Marjorie Skubic, Kathryn Burks, Jie Yu, George Demiris, Brian K. Hensel, Gregory L. Alexander, Zhihai He, Harry W. Tyrer, Marc Hamilton, Jia Lee, and Marybeth Brown

2.1 Importance of Functional Assessment for Older Adults

Functional well-being is a significant factor in the overall health of older people. The World Health Organization advisory group stated almost 40 years ago that the health of older adults was best measured in terms of function [1]. Generally speaking, function as an overall term can be divided into three categories: physical, psychological, and social function [2]. The three components interact closely and contribute to the overall construct of well-being. A comprehensive geriatric functional assessment is usually composed of these components. For example, Nelson and associates interchangeably used terms of function, functional health, and functional status as they conducted a complete functional assessment using separate measures of components, such as physical function, emotional status, role and social function, pain and social support [3].

The purpose of the comprehensive functional assessment among the elderly is to bridge the gap between people's actual abilities and the available resources [4]. A regular functional assessment can help clinicians easily identify older people's changes over time so that effective strategies can be implemented in a timely manner to prevent or reduce severe negative outcomes. Physical function is the key factor of functional assessment, and it is sometimes synonymous with functional status or functioning in current literature. The goal of this section is to examine the meaning of physical function as it relates to the overall functional assessment and to explore the significance of physical function to comprehensive geriatric functional assessment.

Marilyn Rantz
Professor, Sinclair School of Nursing and Family and Community Medicine, S 406 Sinclair School of Nursing, University of Missouri-Columbia, Columbia, MO 65211
e-mail: RantzM@HEALTH.MISSOURI.EDU

From: *Aging Medicine, Eldercare Technology for Clinical Practitioners,*
Edited by: M. Alwan and R. Felder © Humana Press, Totowa, NJ

2.1.1 Physical Function

Physical function is a commonly used term among researchers; however, there are few authors who have provided a clear definition of physical function. One example by Brach and VanSwearingen [5] states that physical function is associated with the ability to perform activities of daily living (ADLs), instrumental activities of daily living (IADLs), and mobility tasks, which are important for independent living without substantial risks of injury. McConnell and colleagues [6] referred to physical function as the degree of dependency in basic ADLs and discussed its importance on elders' quality of life. Similarly, Fitzpatrick et al. [7] regarded physical function as the physical ability to engage in daily activities related to personal care, socially defined roles, and recreational activities. These daily activities could be further classified into ADLs (basic self-care activities that include dressing, bathing, personal hygiene, toileting, walking, eating, etc.), IADLs (activities and skills needed to live independently in the community such as shopping, cooking, housekeeping, and handling finances), basic physical movements, and complex actions [8]. In contrast, Whetstone et al. [9] explained physical function as the dynamic changing status of dependency, difficulty, and preclinical changes across a wide range of activities.

Although most researchers did not specifically define the concept of physical function, their understandings of the term are demonstrated by their choices of measurement instruments. For example, Shimada et al. [10] examined physical function by evaluating subjects' balance, gait, and reaction time. Balance was evaluated by one-leg standing time and the Functional Reach Test (FRT); gait performance was measured by walking speed over a 10-m distance and the equipment of Whole Body Reaction Type-II was utilized to assess reaction time to an auditory stimulus (100 Hz). On the contrary, Furner and associates [11] used participants' self-report of performance on ADLs and IADLs to evaluate physical function. Some researchers choose to combine subjective and objective assessments to provide a comprehensive description of the status of physical function. For instance, subjective questionnaires, such as the physical functioning questionnaire (PFQ) and performance-based tests, which include a 6-min walk test, were used simultaneously to evaluate the status of physical function among a group of cardiac older people [12].

It seems that these authors have different understandings of physical function; however, they are concerned about the same construct. Most authors interpret physical function as people's actual physical performance abilities in simple movements, such as walking and standing, or their self-rated abilities on ADLs and IADLs. Additionally, most agree that the status of physical function at a certain time point in aging process could be affected by some physiological and pathological conditions. Therefore, it seems reasonable to conclude that physical function represents a person's current abilities to participate in daily activities relating to different social roles. Specifically, an older adult's actual performance and self reports in some basic daily life activities, ADLs and IADLs, can reflect the status of physical function.

2.1.2 Significance of Physical Function for Older Adults

An appropriate level of physical function plays a significant role in active and independent living for the elderly, and regular assessments will make early detection and timely intervention possible to maintain reasonable or delay the deterioration of physical function. In the trajectory of aging, a person's quality of life is judged more often by the ability to maintain independence and physical function, than by any medical diagnosis [13]. However, lower level of physical function is also associated with significant negative health outcomes, such as hospitalization, nursing home admission, falls, and dependency [14]. Therefore, the assessment of physical function is not only a key component of functional assessment but an important part of comprehensive geriatric evaluation.

Physical function is closely associated with the other two components of functional assessments, social and psychological function, and some gerontological studies have confirmed such relationships. For example, Cronin-Stubbs and colleagues [15] conducted a population-based longitudinal study during a 6-year period in 3434 community-dwelling older people and found that mild depressive symptoms were associated with an increased risk of becoming physically disabled. Similarly, data from the MacArthur Studies of Successful Aging identified depression as a risk factor for physical disability, which was assessed by ADLs Scale. Results also suggested that depression and physical disability could initiate a spiraling decline in both physical and psychological function [16]. Consequently, clinicians should keep in mind that, while addressing the significance of physical function in gerontological care, social and psychological functions and their interactions should not be overlooked. Additionally, the contribution of pain to physical function and depression cannot be overlooked. Often, pain management is the key to improving physical function in older adults.

Some important clinical implications for elder care could be drawn. First, the assessments of physical function should be comprehensive and individualized. Clinicians should not only be familiar with the knowledge about physical function, but also accurately evaluate an older person's level of physical function on a regular basis. Secondly, because there are close interactions among physical, social, and psychological functions, progressive elder care programs should address physical activity involvement, social and intellectual engagement, and pain management among the elderly.

2.1.3 Common Health Conditions that Affect Functional Abilities

Because physical function significantly impacts the abilities of older adults to maintain independence, developing and implementing strategies to prevent or delay the onset of physical disability is a major priority for clinicians. Identifying contributing risk factors to the deterioration of functional abilities is an important step. This section will explore risk factors for declines of physical function and their close interactions with functional abilities.

The decline in functional abilities is not just dependent on chronological age, but is closely associated with other biological, psychological, and social risk factors [17]. For example, Stuck and associates [18] conducted a meta-analysis of 78 longitudinal studies exploring the risk factors for physical function decline in community-living older adults. Some conditions, such as cognitive impairment, depression, disease burden, poor self-rated health, low level of physical activity, and functional limitation, were identified as contributors with highest strength of evidence. The following sections describe key risk factors relating to health conditions and recent research findings in each area are discussed.

2.1.4 Cognitive Impairment

Cognitive function is an important factor for physical function or the abilities to maintain independence among older adults. Previous gerontological studies have confirmed the association between cognitive impairment and physical function. Greiner and associates [19] investigated the relationship of cognitive function to loss of physical function among a group of elderly Catholic nuns. Results showed that participants with low normal cognitive scores on Mini-Mental State Examination (MMSE) at baseline had twice the risk of losing independence in ADLs at follow-up compared with those with high normal scores. This close relationship between cognitive impairments and functional decline is also identified in other populations, such as non-disabled, community-living older adults and elderly Mexican Americans [20, 21].

Besides MMSE, which is an often used cognitive function instrument in aging studies, Moritz et al. [22] found consistent results utilizing another cognitive assessment tool, Pfeiffer's short portable mental status questionnaire (SPMSQ). This longitudinal study revealed persistent and incidental ADL limitations occurred more frequently in older persons with four or more errors on SPMSQ. The result not only confirmed the relationship between cognitive function and physical abilities in ADLs, but also suggested cognitive impairment might be a significant predictor of the onset of new ADL limitations. Conclusions could be made from these studies that cognitive impairment is an important contributor for declines in physical function and predicts the onset of ADL limitations, using a variety of assessment measures.

Accordingly, some implications can be drawn for geriatric clinicians. They should not only be familiar with cognitive impairment, which acts as a significant risk factor for functional decline, but also be aware of the knowledge that some cognitive functional tests can be used to forecast services needed and to plan interventions to delay the onset of ADL limitations or plan strategies to best deal with the limitations [22].

2.1.5 Depression

Although the prevalence of major depression is relatively small (2%) among older community-living persons, a high percentage (12–15%) of elderly community-dwellers suffer from minor depression or significant clinical depressive symptoms [23]. As a crucial contributor to older persons' well-being and functional status, the detrimental effects of depression on physical function have been investigated in numerous aging studies [24–26].

Penninx and associates [26] conducted a 4-year prospective cohort study exploring the impact of depressive symptoms on changes of physical performance among 1286 older community dwellers. After controlling for other conditions (such as baseline performance score, health status, and socio-demographic factors), they found that high levels of depressive symptoms [assessed by the Center for Epidemiologic Studies Depression Scale (CES-D)], could highly predict decline in physical function. These findings were consistent with research done by Everson-Rose et al. [25] substantiating a strong cross-sectional association between depressive symptoms and overall physical performance. Callahan and colleagues [27] also confirmed previous research findings that older persons with depression (evaluated by CES-D) reported greater functional impairment than those without depressive symptoms. Furthermore, a multi-site randomized clinical trial [24] revealed that effective treatment of depressive symptoms by a collaborative program improves physical function more than usual care.

The close relationship between depression and physical function can shed light on future clinical practice. Attention should be paid to the detrimental effects of depression on declines of physical function. Collaborative eldercare programs should be developed to address depression and interrupt the downward spiral of the deterioration of depression and physical performance.

2.1.6 Lack of Physical Activity

Lack of physical activity is also independently related with a higher risk for declines of physical function [18]. Studies have confirmed relationships between physical activity and functional impairment. For example, Seeman and colleagues [28] found a significant and independent association between better physical function and participation in moderate and/or strenuous exercise activity.

Abundant studies have examined the effects of exercise programs in helping improve physical function and maintain independence. Taylor-Piliae and associates [17] detected that Tai Chi exercise could significantly improve balance, upper and lower body muscular strength, endurance, and flexibility. Similarly, from a randomized and placebo-controlled trial, even among nursing home frail residents, a progressive resistance training was found to impressively increase muscle mass and improve functional performance in gait speed and stair-climbing abilities [29]. Frontera and associates [30] also demonstrated that regular resistance training could significantly promote the strength of extensor and flexor muscles in older partici-pants. It is clear that physiological parameters, such as balance, gait performance, muscular strength, endurance, and flexibility are prerequisites to keep an appro-priate level of physical function [31]. Increasing physical activity through exercise programs, such as Tai Chi and resistance training, can significantly improve physical function.

Another view of improving physical function is to *increase non-exercise physical activity* (NEPA). NEPA involves all forms of physical activity other than exercise. Most of a person's NEPA is associated with ambulation for practical purposes or movements not intended for health, including many forms of "puttering." Examples of NEPA that may be critical for preserving health and vitality include the thousands of light movements people associate with an independent and vibrant lifestyle, such as vacuuming, dusting, walking across the room to manually change the television channel, or adjust the blinds. Total energy expenditure is low in aging adults primarily because of less activity or NEPA, not a lower basal metabolic rate [32,33], and more time spent in sedentary activities involving sitting [34]. People over the age of 65 years take almost one-half as many steps per day as younger people. Remarkably, 20% of those aged above 65 years take less than 1000 steps per day, whereas only approximately 1% of middle-aged people less than 65 years take this few steps [35]. Taken together, these and other studies of aging adults with preclinical disability [36] have led to the belief that there is a vicious cycle linking inactivity with metabolic disorders and loss of mobility.

An emerging paradigm of great interest to the exercise physiology research community relates to how simply sitting instead of NEPA leads to increased risk for chronic diseases; the term coined for this new paradigm has been called "inactivity physiology" [37]. Simply put, the time spent standing in any weight-bearing activity (even NEPA) portends to be a determinant of multiple functional and disease end-points relevant to successful aging. Low levels of high-density lipoprotein (HDL) cholesterol are associated with functional disability in the elderly [38]. In addition, bone health is related with the time one sits or stands [39–41].

Epidemiological correlations have associated daily sitting time with metabolic syndrome (low HDL cholesterol, high plasma triglycerides, hypertension, body fat, and insulin resistance or glucose intolerance [42–44]). For each hour less of daily television watching, there was a 12–26% reduction in the incidence of the metabolic syndrome [43]. The ill effect of sitting was independent of whether the person was engaged in traditional exercise [43, 45]. There are mechanistic explanations and interventional studies in animals for those associations. Com-ponents of the metabolic syndrome, diabetes, and cardiovascular disease have each been linked in large part to an enzyme called lipoprotein lipase (LPL). The inactivity found during aging is associated with significantly lower levels of LPL [46, 47]. The function of LPL is strongly suppressed to only 5% of normal levels after reduced standing and is preventable by increased standing and NEPA [48, 49]. NEPA measurements and interventions in the elderly or functionally impaired could thus be especially important to improve physical function.

2.1.7 Other Factors Affecting Functional Abilities

Some other factors, such as co-morbidities, few social contacts, poor self-perceived health, smoking, and vision impairment, have also been identified in current literature as strongly related to physical function decline [18]. Higher body weight has been recognized as an important risk factor for lower every day physical functioning [50]. Other researchers have also revealed that factors such as positive motivation and appropriate social roles can positively influence physical function in performance-based tests [51].

2.1.8 Summary, Functional Abilities

As an indispensable component of independent living while aging, physical function is and has always been the integral focus of clinical geriatric care. Some common health conditions, such as cognitive impairment, depression, and a lack of physical activity, which significantly contribute to the decline of physical function, have been reviewed. These significant contributing factors for declines of physical function should be identified regularly to prevent or delay severe deterioration and should be sufficiently addressed in comprehensive care programs.

Understanding the significance of physical function and risk factors for functional decline can help those interested in technology as a way to help older adults maintain or regain function. Technology should enhance the on-going assessment of physical function that is a major focus of clinicians. It is our belief that technology holds the capacity to enhance clinical effectiveness by early detection of changes in function, alerting clinicians and providing functional assessment information about functional performance of older adults in their care.

2.2 Common Measures of Functional Assessment

Physical function is the basis of overall well-being among the elders, and its accurate and sensitive measurement is a vital component in gerontological care. A variety of reliable and valid physical function instruments exist in current literature. There are three main kinds of instruments: self-report and proxy report, performance-based tests, and objective laboratory tests. This section will explore each category individually. Representative measures of each group will be discussed, and their characteristics will be examined and compared. Finally, the appropriate use of these instruments will be discussed.

2.2.1 Self-Report and Proxy Report

Self-report and proxy report assessments focus on self or proxy perception of physical function [14]. They are both relatively easy to administer and usually require little instruction for participants. Because self-report assessments are completed by subjects themselves, information about the overall perception of the individual regarding their health status and ability to perform certain activities are available [14]. In contrast, proxy reports are executed by family members or health professionals based on their observation of subjects' performance on certain tasks.

Measures that determine subjects' difficulty in performing ADLs and IADLs are often employed in various studies to monitor the changes in physical function. For example, there are direct ADLs and IADLs indices [52], as well as measures such as the functional status questionnaire (FSQ) that include specific sections addressing these aspects of physical function [53]. Similarly, the Western Ontario and McMaster Universities Osteoarthritis Index (WOMAC), a disease-specific measure, includes questions that focus on the subject's ability to perform ADLs and IADLs [54–56].

Assessment of pain and pain management strategies are often overlooked in self report and proxy report of physical function. Self report of pain and pain management strategies can be readily completed in simple perception-rating scales such as those recommended in research-based clinical practice guidelines [57]. As physical function is assessed, pain and pain management strategies should also be solicited.

2.2.2 Performance-Based Tests

Performance-based tests of physical function are ones in which subjects are asked to actually perform some specific tasks or activities and are evaluated using standardized criteria [13]. These tests are much more objective and psychometrically sound than self-reports and can offer more sensitive and accurate information.

Instead of measuring the whole construct of physical function, most performance tests are divided into subcategories and evaluate individual components of physical function, such as balance, gait, flexibility, and endurance [14]. Accordingly, the status of physical function can be drawn from overall performance on all or some of these subcategories. For example, Toraman and Sahin [58] used a Functional Fitness Battery to assess physical function. Components of this battery include lower and upper body strength, body flexibility, aerobic endurance, agility, and dynamic balance. Aerobic endurance and lower body strength are measured by simple activities, such as 6-min walk and chair-stand [58]. Similarly, Kenny et al. [59] used the short physical performance battery test (SPPB) to examine the efficacy of vitamin D supplementation among elders. Physical function in this battery is assessed from subjects' performance on rising from a chair, static balance, a 6-foot walk, the time up-and-go test, and the timed supine-to-stand test. Rekeneire and associates [60] also utilized a series of performance-based tests to study physical function. In this study, the timed repeated chair stand was used to assess lower extremity strength and 400 m as well as 2-min walk were used to measure endurance. Subjects' status of physical function was reflected from performance on these tests.

Table 2.1 Selected Instruments Comparisons

Instrument name	Author, Citation	Concepts measured	Scoring	Procedures, administration time	Limitation	Strength
Timed up and go test (TUG) (61)	Podsiadlo, D., Richardson, S. (1991). The timed "Up & Go": A test of basic functional mobility for frail elderly person. *Journal of the American Geriatrics Society* 39:142–8.	Physical mobility.	Time the whole performance. <20 sec: independently mobile of basic transfers; [20, 30]: varies in physical function and further assessment is needed; >30 sec: dependence on help for basic transfers and risk of falls.	Individuals stand up from a standard arm chair (approximate height of 46 cm), walk 3 m, turn, walk back to the chair and sit down again. 10 minutes.	It could not measure changes of functional mobility in either the freely mobile or the very dependent populations, although it could identify them.	It is easy and quick to administer and requires little training or equipment. An objective, reliable, and valid test for quantifying functional mobility.
Physical performance test (PPT) [62].	Reuben, D.B., Siu, A.L. (1990). An objective measure of physical function of elderly outpatients: the physical performance test. *Journal of the American Geriatrics Society* 38:1105–12.	Upper fine and coarse motor function, balance, mobility, coordination, and endurance.	Time individual tasks. The maximum score is 36 for the nine-item test and 28 for the seven-item test.	Nine-item scale: write a sentence, simulate eating, turn 360 degrees, put on and remove a jacket, lift a book, and put it on a shelf, pick up a penny from the floor, a 50-foot walk test and climb stairs. Seven-item scale: not include the stairs. 10 min.	Cannot differentiate from unmotivated from incapable persons and tasks included may not be complete measures of functional status.	Valid, reliable, and easy to administer.

(continued)

Table 2.1 (continued)

Instrument name	Author, Citation	Concepts measured	Scoring	Procedures, administration time	Limitation	Strength
Tinetti assessment tool (63)	Tinetti, M.E. (1986). Performance-oriented assessment of mobility problems in elderly patients. *Journal of the American Geriatrics Society* 34:119–26.	Balance and gait.	Maximum total score is 28. <19: a high risk for falls; [19,24]: a risk for falls.	It is a task performance test. Participants are asked to perform specific maneuvers about balance and gait. 10–15 minutes.	The observations are crude and more variability among individuals could not be found.	A simple and practical performance test. Reliable and sensitive to significant changes used in normal daily living.
Berg balance scale (64)	Berg, K., Wood-Dauphinee, S., Williams, J.I., Gayton, D. (1989). Measuring balance in the elderly: Preliminary development of an instrument. *Physiotherapy Canada* 41(6):304–11.	Balance.	Maximum score is 56. <20: wheelchair bound; [21,40]: walking with assistance; [41,56]: independent.	14 performance-based measures. 10–15 min.	The observations are crude and small changes could hardly be detected.	Objective, valid, and reliable balance measure. Easy to administer and safe for older people.

Four widely used performance-based assessments are summarized in Table 2.1: Timed up and go (TUG) test [61], physical performance test (PPT) [62], Tinetti assessment tool [63], and Berg balance scale [64]. Specific information, such as subscales, scoring criteria, strength, and limitation concerning each instrument are identified and compared.

2.2.3 Laboratory Testing

Physical function and physical fitness are often used interchangeably; therefore, physical function can also be measured in objective laboratory tests that focus on physical fitness. For example, Rejeski et al. [12] combined an objective laboratory test of metabolic equivalent (MET) level with self-report questionnaire and a 6-min walk test to assess physical function in the elderly. Because physical fitness laboratory tests usually require expensive equipment and specially trained technicians, they are not practical for routine physical function assessments.

2.2.4 Summary, Common Measures of Functional Assessment

Appropriate measurement of physical function in the elderly requires multifaceted measurement that addresses the specific attributes of this population especially the close association of physical function with health status [14]. Three main kinds of measurements, self and proxy reports, performance-based tests, and laboratory tests are discussed. In addition, the four most widely used measurement tools are compared. Geriatric clinicians and researchers are encouraged to use a multifaceted approach to measure physical function by combining subjective measures, such as self or proxy reports and objective instruments, such as performance-based tests.

2.3 Overview of Home-Based Eldercare Technologies to Promote and Assess Function

Recent advances in sensor and information technologies have made an important contribution to the care of elderly people. A wide variety of technologies and devices have been developed to promote and support their independent and safe living. In general, these technologies can be classified into two basic categories: assistive devices and monitoring and response systems. These technologies and devices are often coupled together into a smart home environment so as to provide an integrated support for independent living of elderly people.

2.3.1 Assistive Devices

Functional decline in mobility makes it hard for older adults to operate many small appliances at home. At the Georgia Institute of Technology, computer vision researchers have prototyped the Gesture Pendant as a wearable device to control a variety of home appliances through simple hand gestures [65]. A recent study shows that computerized devices are able to help a person with severe dementia complete some ADLs, such as hand washing or using recorded voices for cueing [66]. For people with severe memory impairment, the technologies developed at the University of Michigan are able to remind an older person about his or her ADLs [67]. Medication compliance devices have also been developed to remind an older adult to take medication at the right time and in the right dose [68].

2.3.2 Monitoring and Response System

Individuals with mobility, cognitive, and sensory impairments may not be able to recognize and avoid unsafe conditions, or ask for help during a crisis situation; monitoring systems with sensors can help satisfy this need. Floor vibration monitors have been developed at the University of Virginia to detect possible falls of older adults [69]. Technologies are available to monitor ADL tasks in the home using a variety of sensing technologies. Sensors and switches attached to various objects, or optical and audio sensors embedded in the environment, are used to detect which task a person is performing [70,71]. The University of Virginia In-Home Monitoring System that uses a combination of wireless motion sensors to detect movement in areas of a person's living space can differentiate such ADL activities as showering or meal preparation. Inference of the ADL activities is done in a rule-based approach and has been validated in a community home with a healthy volunteer subject keeping detailed PDA-based time-stamped field notes [72, 73]. These same researchers have also developed a bed sensor for monitoring qualitative pulse and respiration, as well as sleep restlessness [74], which can provide basic indicators of health.

TigerPlace is an innovative independent living environment of 33 apartments built and operated by Americare of Sikeston, MO, USA, in affiliation with the University of Missouri (MU) Sinclair School of Nursing as a special facility where residents can truly age in place and never fear being moved to a traditional nursing home unless they choose to do so. With care provided by Sinclair Home Care and the TigerCare wellness center with registered nurse care coordination services, residents receive preventative and early illness recognition assistance that have markedly improved their lives. Links with MU students, faculty, and nearly every school or college on campus enrich the lives of the students and residents of Tiger-Place. Research projects are encouraged and residents who choose to participate are enjoying helping with developing cutting technology to help other seniors' age in place. The Aging in Place Project at MU required legislation in 1999 and 2001 to be fully realized. Sinclair Home Care is an innovative home health agency initiated by the Sinclair School of Nursing specifically *to help older adults age in place in the environment of their choice.*

The residents of TigerPlace have embraced technology research to help them and others in the future age in place. Many of them are participating in on-going research with developing sensor technology to measure and interpret ADLs, detect falls, and early detection of illness or changes in chronic health conditions. As researchers with funding from the National Science Foundation and Administration on Aging, we are grateful to their willingness to help us as we pioneer this important area of elder care and the development of technology to help them improve and maintain function as they age in place in their homes.

At TigerPlace we have installed the University of Virginia monitoring system with bed, motion, and stove sensors wirelessly connected to a computer that sends the event information to a server. Counting the events provides useful information that indicates resident movement or absence of movement. In a sense, this provides continuous functional assessment because the resident's actions trigger events that are collected by the sensor and counted. The events are organized into a display of counts of the various sensors over a short period of time; typically the most convenient is an hour or several hours. Moreover, sensor firings could be grouped and activities could be inferred. The bed sensor activity counts per day are shown in Fig. 2.1; using daily graphs can reveal trends over time that may indicate changes in resident physical condition. From the bed sensor, greater activity may be due to a variety of factors including incorrect medicine dosage and impending change in health. By examining the data, a picture emerges of activities of the individual. By relating the histogram data for the resident to resident's comments about those events potential causes of events can be interpreted.

In the display of bed restlessness data in Fig. 2.1, a dramatic change in resident condition can be seen. This particular resident had a heart attack around December 20. For several days following the event, the resident was in the hospital and no events appeared. After returning, significantly higher restlessness levels indicate health-related problems. In later graphs in February, after the problems were addressed, the subject's restlessness levels returned to low levels similar to the graphs before the heart attack.

Clearly, this technology is potentially useful to health care providers. First, it provides additional information to health care providers by displaying a quick indication of the resident's well being, and possible deviations from their individual norm. It can provide loved ones access to activity information of their important elder family member (if the elder agrees) using relatively well-established communication systems such as web access. The data provide a longitudinal record of activity that can be examined for changes.

By relating the changes in sensor data to specific events of resident activity, a health care provider can obtain a picture of specific functional decline. Once identified, functional decline may be minimized or halted by appropriate interventions such as physical therapy, changes in medications, or others. Early detection and intervention by health care providers can extend the level of function of a resident and possibly even improve it. Modeling individual elder's activities with advanced computational intelligence techniques can enable interpretation of the baseline activity of individuals and alert health care providers of potential changes from baseline. Significant deviations from an individual's norm may indicate changes that require action.

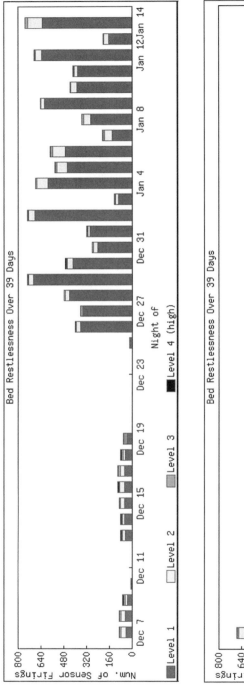
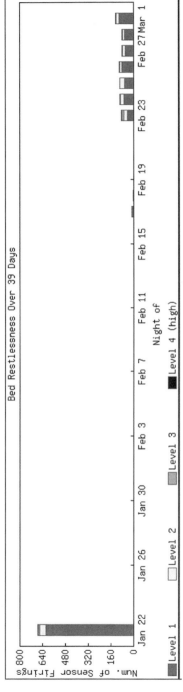

Fig. 2.1 Bed Restlessness Data Graph, showing different levels of restlessness from level 1 (least restless) to level 4 (most restless)

2.3.3 Smart Home Technologies

A smart home is a home that is able to proactively change its environment to provide services that promote an independent lifestyle for elderly users. Honeywell's Independent Lifestyle Assistant (ILSA) program is targeted at developing an intelligent home automation system to enable elders to live and function safely at home [75, 76]. The Living laboratory at MIT uses a portable kit of tape-on sensors and small switches to detect the movement of objects. They also studied how people respond to new proactive technologies [77]. In the Aware Home project at the Georgia Institute of Technology, a house with two identical independent living spaces is built for controlled experiments with technologies [78]. In France, a smart home called PROSAFE has been designed. Devices and sensors identify abnormal behavior that can be interpreted as an accident and collect representative data on a person's nocturnal and daily activity. The experimental room has been designed to accommodate patients with Alzheimer's disease. It is equipped with a set of infrared motion sensors connected to either a wireless or a wired network.

Realizing that visual information is very important in activity monitoring and analysis, researchers have developed various video camera systems and vision-processing algorithms for eldercare. In the Aware Home project at Georgia Institute of Technology, video cameras are used in a research laboratory to capture images of resident's daily activities, and a user-friendly interface, called Digital Family Portrait, is developed to efficiently visualize the activity data and resident's health status [78, 79]. In the CareMedia project at Carnegie Mellon University, a video camera system is developed to monitor patients' activity in nursing homes. Coupled with other types of sensor information and medical data, the video information is used to study the behavioral patterns of patients [80].

The University of Virginia In-Home Monitoring System has been installed in another assisted living setting ($n = 15$) and in another independent living setting ($n = 25$) (other than TigerPlace). In both settings, evaluations of Satisfaction with Life were obtained from the participating residents and modified Caregiver Strain Indexes as well as Caregiver Burden Interviews were obtained from the professional and informal caregivers [73, 81–83]. The only significant changes were that Satisfaction with Life improved in assisted living residents, and there was a statistically significant increase in informal care-giving but no increase in burden or strain. These same monitoring systems were installed in the homes of 13 home care clients [84] with similar results; clients had better perceived quality of life and informal care-givers had a perceived reduction in strain. From these preliminary results, it appears that using technology to monitor activity may have positive effects for elders in all three settings as well as some benefit for informal care givers. Cost-benefit in a sample of 21 assisted living residents has also been examined over a 3-month period as compared with a matched group by these same researchers with a significant reduction in health care costs such as hospital days, emergency room visits, and other primary care costs [85].

2.4 End User Interface Design for Functional Assessment Systems

Home-based functional assessment systems need to enable the processing and efficient display of information resulting from the sensor components. One of the challenges with the capturing of functional assessment, activity levels, and sleep patterns through sensor or other systems is the presentation of information to health care providers in a timely manner and with a display that does not burden providers with complex or redundant information but at the same time highlights situations that require attention or emergencies.

It is a widely accepted notion that user participation in the design and development of information systems increases the likelihood of successful implementation and utilization of these systems [86, 87]. Involvement of end users in system design is likely to result in increased user satisfaction [88], and an increase in the perception of usefulness of the application by the end user [89, 90]. Lack of communication and collaboration, on the contrary, between end users and designers is often linked to failure of information technology (IT) implementations [91].

In many cases, system failure is attributed to exclusion of end users from the system and interface design of monitoring systems. Organizations or agencies face the challenge to select the appropriate timing and extent of end user involvement in various phases of system development given, in many cases, limited resources and time constraints. Thus, understanding the nature of user participation and its implications on the utilization and ultimately the success of a system provides a useful roadmap for the implementation of both small- and large-scale applications.

2.4.1 Clinicians as End Users

In the TigerPlace project, nurses are one of the main user groups of the monitoring system. Additional user groups include residents, family members, and informal caregivers. To determine nurses' preferences and expectations of user interfaces that will enable the processing and efficient display of information resulting from the smart home components, we conducted focus group sessions with four gerontology nurses and one social worker [92]. The session was facilitated by a member of the TigerPlace research team. The focus group protocol included questions about participants' preferences in accessing patient-related data, their critique of suggested interfaces, and additional questions about types of display and alerts that will be useful in monitoring and caring for senior residents.

Specific examples of interfaces were displayed and comments were solicited in terms of advantages and disadvantages. Three of these examples were discussed in greater detail as they were perceived as essential to the display of activity levels and sleep patterns. Hard copies and large displays of the examples of user interfaces were provided to allow participants a careful examination before the discussion. The focus group facilitator followed a protocol of questions and took notes. Descriptive cues, examples, and explanations were provided, when necessary. Data codes were generated by using the data collected. The goal of the qualitative content analysis was a summary of the information gleaned from the analyses of data.

The clinicians who participated stated that non-emergency data sets should be available on a secure website allowing for providers to access them at their own discretion. Emergency alerts triggered by the system indicating a situation that requires immediate attention should be sent in *multiple formats*, such as email messages, pager messages, phone calls etc. The discussion whether this information should become part of the patient's medical record did not reach consensus. Some clinicians stated that that should be the case, whereas others expressed the concern that smart home technologies should move beyond the experimental phase before the datasets they produce become part of a legal document. Most participants stated that the interface should allow users to enter interpretations and other notes and provide a platform for communication with other health care providers.

Visual summaries and *overall trends* were perceived as very useful in managing large data sets. Participants showed preference for *interactive visual displays* that would allow zoom-in and zoom-out features, and ability to click for more information or enter comments. Furthermore, all participants agreed that they would like the interface to provide a "*print-version*" of the datasets so that they can easily create a hard copy for further review or archiving purposes. This study also highlighted the emphasis that clinicians place as end users on *internal* and *external consistency* of the interfaces and *interoperability* of this application with other applications and, specifically, the electronic medical record software (regardless of whether these datasets end up becoming part of the record system). All participants pointed out the need for consistency in choice of colors and symbols.

2.4.2 Interfaces between IT Systems

In a recent qualitative study using key informant interviews and focus group methods, 12 long-term care health care providers, administrators, and IT developers explored the use of advanced electronic technologies as it affects patient care, clinical support, and administrative activities [93]. The most important thread of information about IT sophistication emerging from these discussions regarded the need for more advanced interface development for IT systems to enhance system integration and connectivity. There was a recognized need for development of interfaces that support communication between different IT systems in order to build common data repositories and data warehouses. Interface operability was recognized as a vitally important issue.

Interfaces are important because they allow for the exchange of vital clinical information and contribute to the formation of relational databases that can combine distinct datasets into powerful reporting tools. Interfaces reduce the duplicative work required to keep separate IT systems current and facilitate a safer environment through more consistent data entry, faster retrieval of information, and improved reliability of data sources.

An important aspect of IT sophistication that is related to interface development is the usability of IT systems. Functional sophistication and integration of clinical decision support can be positively or negatively affected by the users' perceptions, accuracy of information input into the system, and the specificity of information guiding users' decisions. Increased levels of IT support and training personnel can improve usability, contribute to the design of sophisticated systems, keep the technology up and running smoothly, and are important for maintaining connections with users of IT. For clinical end users, integration of data with other clinical data sources is essential for rapid decision support that will ultimately improve quality of care for older adults.

2.4.3 Patients and Family Members as End Users

As stated earlier, end users include not only the clinicians and health care providers but also the actual residents or patients and their family members. A large portion of patients requiring functional assessment services are elderly and in some cases have functional limitations because of aging and/or their diagnosis. The Telecommunications Industry Association [94] describes a functional limitation as a "...reduced sensory, cognitive or motor capability associated with human aging, temporary injury, or permanent disability that prevents a person from communicating, working, playing or simply functioning in an environment where other people in the population can function." Although many argue that the Internet and advanced telecommunication technologies have the potential to empower patients and even revolutionize the process of health care delivery, the fastest growing segment of the US population (i.e., people over the age of 50 years) are at a disadvantage because software and hardware designers often fail to consider them as a potential user group.

Usability and accessibility issues are important quality criteria for web-based interventions, but are frequently ignored by designers and evaluators. The design of a usable web-based information system that will allow residents to monitor their own functional assessment data becomes a challenge when it targets users inexperienced with the technology and with possible functional limitations. Therefore, systems targeting older adults should have reached a high level of functional accessibility [95] and undergone rigorous usability tests. Several design considerations can be taken into account when developing systems for the elderly or other populations with functional limitations.

2.4.4 Privacy and Confidentiality

When designing systems that allow web access to patients, family members, and health care providers, the issues of privacy and confidentiality of individual health information have to be addressed. Information privacy is the patient's right to control the use and dissemination of information that relates to them. Confidentiality is a tool for protecting the patients' privacy. Thus, system designers need to take into consideration that the patient has the right to allow family members to access information about their activity level but may also choose not to. When discussing privacy, issues related to the video- and/or audio-recording and maintenance of tapes, the storage and transmission of still images, and other patient record data must be examined, and efforts must be undertaken to address them to the fullest extent possible. The transmission of information over communication lines such as phone lines, satellite, or other channels, is associated with concerns of possible privacy violations. An additional concern in some cases is the presence of technical staff assisting with the transmission procedure that could be perceived as a loss of privacy by the patients. Patients often are unfamiliar with the technical infrastructure and operation of the equipment which can lead to misperceptions of the possibilities of privacy violation.

Furthermore, ownership of and access to data must be addressed. In many web-based applications in home care, patients record monitoring data and transmit them daily to a web server owned and maintained by a private third party that allows providers to log in and access their patients' data. This type of application calls for discussion and definition of the issue of data ownership and patients' access rights to parts or all of their records.

2.4.5 Interdisciplinary Approach to System Design

An interdisciplinary approach is essential to design a home that is flexible and responsive to the needs and limitations of the residents. The value of interdisciplinary teams is not a new concept in gerontology. Such teams overcome the problems of the traditional health care organizational model, which reinforces functional specialties and silos of expertise. The interdisciplinary team approach promotes integrated and coordinated care for older adults so that all participants in the care-delivery process are focused on the older adult rather than their professional specialty. During both the design and the development phases of a smart home, experts from different disciplines need to be included. As Rogers [96] points out, we need to shift from a model of "technological determinism," namely that technology itself should be the impetus for change, to a model of the social construction of technology where technology is influenced by societal norms and needs.

The success of functional assessment systems or smart homes in general will depend on the level of compliance with universal design principles that are holistic and inclusive [97]. Many of the challenges that older adults face, whether functional or cognitive limitations, have been traditionally addressed by the utilization of mechanical adaptive devices, which allow the user to adequately function in their environment, but not necessarily actively participate in it. The use of adaptive and assistive technology that can be installed in the home environment has the potential to not only support but also enable and empower individual users.

2.5 End-User Perceptions of Home-Based Technologies for Functional Assessment

It is axiomatic that end-users' perceptions of an "elective" home-based technology for functional assessment are central to whether they accept and adopt it. Such perceptions contribute to, possibly determine, success in both the implementation and the sustained use of these technologies. Ideally, end-users of such information-based health-monitoring technologies work in partnership with their health care providers to "co-produce" the quality of their care and, ultimately, their health [98, 99]. Optimal management of chronic disease and functional decline demands such an approach.

Measures of end-user acceptance of, and satisfaction with, informatics technologies are often focused on an application's usability or user-friendliness and, for users with physical or cognitive limitations, its accessibility. Although these factors are important in other eldercare applications, they do not directly impact end-users of passive sensor monitoring devices like those at TigerPlace (except in the informational user reports these devices generate). A broader set of measures is necessary, especially for user perceptions of these technologies in the home environment.

People have different expectations of the personal space in their home or residence than of public spaces. We view health care monitoring and assessment technologies applied to us as a patient in a hospital (e.g., cardiac telemetry) differently than when they are applied in our home. Negative feelings associated with dependence may be especially strong in the home setting. Ruddick [100] explains how a person's "sense of self often changes with place, especially with place of residence (p. 20)." He goes on to compare the hospital patient's "sick self" to his or her self at home—"one's defining, natural, or 'telic' place (p. 20)."

The home telehealth literature, which includes functional assessment applications, recommends that such technologies be designed and implemented to minimize their obtrusiveness or intrusiveness to users in their home environments. However, these terms are not explicitly defined or consistently used [101]. In response, based on a review of the literature, Hensel et al. [102] proposed a model of obtrusiveness (Figure 2.2) with eight dimensions and twenty-two sub-categories. In this model, "obtrusiveness" in home-based technologies for functional assessment is an umbrella construct inclusive of "intrusiveness" and is defined as "a summary evaluation by the user based on characteristics or effects associated with the technology that are perceived as undesirable and physically and/or psychologically prominent (p. 20)." Although this model still must be validated, it provides a framework within which to examine older adults' perceptions of these technologies.

The model was developed to capture potential obtrusiveness across a comprehensive range of eldercare technologies, including those used in functional assessment. Some dimensions and categories may be more important to users of a passive sensor-based assessment system, such as at TigerPlace, than to users of different types of eldercare technologies. For example, within the physical dimension, users of a remotely monitored oxygen system may perceive it as obtrusive because they

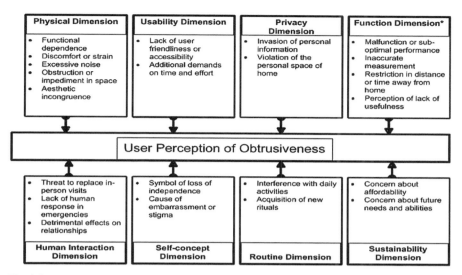

Fig. 2.2 Model of Obtrusiveness in Home-Based Technologies for Functional Assessment (reprinted with permission from the *Journal of the American Medical Informatics Association*) *Function dimension refers to function of the technology.

are functionally dependent on the technology. Conversely, TigerPlace residents are not, in a direct sense, functionally dependent on the sensors.

Consistent with this example, no participants of focus groups across two studies [103,104] prospectively evaluated the TigerPlace sensors as potentially obtrusive because of physical *functional dependence*. On the contrary, comments were found in the focus group transcripts of each study expressing concerns that fit in the physical dimension subcategories of *obstruction or spatial impediment* and *aesthetic incongruence*. There were two dimensions in which concerns in each of the two studies included every subcategory: privacy and self-concept. Privacy was generally viewed in balance with health needs: greater health needs may mean sacrificing some privacy in terms of personal information and access to the personal space of home. Concerns expressed within the self-concept dimension reinforced that independence in relation to this technology is important not only in physical terms but also in psychological and even social terms (i.e., What will others think?).

In a third study [105] using focus groups, which broadly explored perceptions about these types of "smart home" technologies and was held before the selection of specific TigerPlace sensors, participants similarly voiced concerns about privacy. Consistent with the other studies, privacy concerns for some were heightened surrounding the use of cameras, although these apprehensions lessened when it was explained that video could be "anonymized" such that only gross movements, not individual features, would be depicted. Also consistent with the other studies, this earlier study found a focus on the function of technology in emergency response, especially in detection and response to falls.

Next steps at TigerPlace include examining the retrospective perceptions of residents who have sensors installed in their apartments. Potential future research questions include whether perceptions change to include the preventative utility of sensor monitors in detecting health problems earlier and thus facilitating earlier treatment. Another area of potentially fruitful research is the role of end-user control (e.g., the ability to turn off a sensor) in mediating perceived obtrusiveness, especially in the dimension of privacy.

An important qualitative finding across all three focus group studies was a general openness and favorability toward technologies that can help older persons maintain their independence. Moreover, simply because aspects of a technology are perceived as obtrusive by an individual does not necessarily mean he or she will not use it. Other factors such as perceived need undoubtedly greatly influence this decision. We do not know the generalized relationship between perceptions of obtrusiveness as defined in the dimensions and subcategories of the conceptual model and the adoption of a technology. Describing this relationship would necessitate a validated and reliable instrument for measuring obtrusiveness, applied in multiple large studies across different settings and populations. Obtrusiveness is conceptually defined as a "subjective" "summary evaluation," which may be based on "a number of characteristics or effects associated with the technology or one . . . that is especially important . . . to the user [102] (p. 22)."

Even though it is in an early stage of development, the model appears to provide a useful conceptual framework, with seventeen of the twenty-two categories found in at least one of the three focus group studies. Of course, different populations will emphasize different concerns. Participants in these focus group studies were relatively independent and lived within the monitored environment of an independent living facility.

This section intended to stress the importance of end-user perceptions of a functional assessment technology to their adoption of it and ultimate satisfaction with it. To assist in this assessment, a framework is provided to explore end-user perceptions of obtrusiveness of individual applications of these technologies.

2.6 Challenges for Technology Experts to Implement Functional Assessment Technologies in the Real World

There is remaining work to be done. It is not yet clear that data that are collected are complete in the sense of capturing functional assessment. It is unclear whether all the data that are needed or that all the events that are needed can be collected. It seems that activity of humans easily outstrips the ability of sensors to detect all the details that are needed for interpretation. There appears to be no perfect and specific set of sensors to capture all activity. Additionally, correlating activity with multiple sensors may not be sufficient and computational techniques may not adequately describe the activity nor sufficiently compute it for interpretation.

A major concern is that some technologies may be seen as obtrusive. Clearly, video technology requires means of assuring the residents that their images will be protected. Although video coupled with other imaging modalities have great usefulness as monitoring sensing systems, that usefulness must be tempered with the need to make the technology as unobtrusive as possible. Privacy is an important issue and one we believe *must be controlled by the individual resident.* Clearly, the resident must decide who sees their activity information and who does not. As long as technology is in the research stage, the institutional review board and human subject protection policies provide mechanisms to assure privacy. However, when the technology is released to the public for general use, it must be the elder resident who determines who gets what data. This concern will become acute as the resident's functional and cognitive abilities decline. Advanced planning will need to consider technologies and information just as treatment decisions are made in advance for medical care.

Technology has huge potential for the health and function of elders. It must be used wisely and always from the perspective of improving their independence, dignity, and function. Focus groups and interviews with elder users of technology and sensitivity to their needs by not only health care providers but also those developing the technology will go a long way to minimizing obtrusiveness of technology. The acceptance of technology by both health care providers and elders will help realize the promise that elders will achieve more independence and higher quality of life, and providers and loved ones will have more ready, useful, and accurate information about function and health status.

References

1. World Health Organization. (1959). The public health aspects of the aging of the population. Copenhagen.
2. Sehy, Y.B., Williams, M.P. (1999). Functional assessment. In Stone, J.T., Wyman, J.F., Salisbury, S.A. (Eds). *Clinical Gerontological Nursing: A guide to advanced practice* (2nd ed.) W.B. Saunders Company, pp. 175–202.
3. Nelson, E.C., et al. (1998). Dartmouth COOP functional health assessment charts: Brief measures for clinical practice (The Dartmouth College COOP Project). Retrieved 11 September 2005 from http://www.dartmouth.edu/~ coopproj/index.html
4. Williams, T.F., Williams, M. (1982). Assessment of the elderly for long-term care. *Journal of the American Geriatrics Society* 30(1):71–5.
5. Brach, J.S., VanSwearingen, J.M. (2002). Physical impairment and disability: Relationship to performance of activities of daily living in community-dwelling older men. *Physical Therapy* 82(8):752–61.
6. McConnell, E.S., et al. (2003). Natural history of change in physical function among long-stay nursing home residents. *Nursing Research* 52(2):119–26.
7. Fitzpatrick, J.J., et al. (2000). *Geriatric Nursing Research Digest.* Springer Publishing Company, NY.
8. Katz, S., et al. (1963). Studies of illness in the aged: The index of ADL: A standardized measure of biological and psychological function. *Journal of the American Medical Association.* 185(12):914–9.
9. Whetstone, L.M., et al. (2001). The Physical Functioning Inventory: A procedure for assessing physical function in adults. *Journal of Aging and Health* 13(4):467–93.

10. Shimada, H., et al. (2004). New intervention program for preventing falls among frail elderly people: The effects of perturbed walking exercise using a bilateral separated treadmill. *American Journal of Physical Medicine & Rehabilitation* 83(7):493–9.

11. Furner, S.E., et al. (2004). A co-twin control study of physical function in elderly African American women. *Journal of Aging and Health* 16(1):28–43.

12. Rejeski, W.J., et al. (2002). Older adults in cardiac rehabilitation: A new strategy for enhancing physical function. *Medicine and Science in Sports and Exercise* 34(11):1705–13.

13. Guralnik, J.M., et al. (1989). Physical performance measures in aging research. *Journal of Gerontology* 44(5): M141–6.

14. Painter, P., Stewart, A.L., Carey, S. (1999). Physical functioning: Definitions, measurement, and expectations. *Advanced Renal Replacement Therapy* 6:110–23.

15. Cronin-Stubbs, D., et al. (2000). Six-year effect of depressive symptoms on the course of physical disability in community-living older adults. *Archives of Internal Medicine* 160(13):3074–80.

16. Bruce, M.L., et al. (1994). The impact of depressive symptomatology on physical disability: MacArthur Studies of Successful Aging. *American Journal of Public Health* 84(11):1796–9.

17. Taylor-Piliae, R.E., et al. (2006). Improvement in balance, strength, and flexibility after 12 weeks of Tai Chi exercise in ethnic Chinese adults with cardiovascular disease risk factors. *Alternative Therapies* 12(2):50–8.

18. Stuck, A.E., et al. (1998). Risk factors for functional status decline in community-living elderly people: A systematic literature review. *Social and Science Medicine* 48:445–69.

19. Greiner, P.A., Snowdon, D.A., Schmitt, F.A. (1996). The loss of independence in activities of daily living: The role of low normal cognitive function in elderly nuns. *American Journal of Public Health* 86(1):62–6.

20. Grill, T.M., et al. (1996). Impairments in physical performance and cognitive status as predisposing factors for functional dependence among nondisabled older persons. *Journals of Gerontology Series A: Biological Sciences and Medical Sciences* 51A(6):M283–8.

21. Raji, M.A., et al. (2002). The interaction of cognitive and emotional status on subsequent physical functioning in older Mexican Americans: Findings from the Hispanic Established Population for the Epidemiologic Study of the Elderly. *Journals of Gerontology Series A: Biological Sciences and Medical Sciences* 57A(10):M678–82.

22. Moritz, D.J., Kasl, S.V., Berkman, L.F. (1995). Cognitive functioning and the incidence of limitations in activities of daily living in an elderly community sample. *American Journal of Epidemiology* 141(1):41–9.

23. Beekman, A.T., et al. (1995). Major and minor depression in later life: A study of prevalence and risk factors. *Journal of Affective Disorders* 36:65–75.

24. Callahan, C.M., et al. (2005). Treatment of depression improved physical performance in older adults. *Journal of American Geriatrics Society* 53:367–73.

25. Everson-Rose, S.A., et al. (2005). Do depressive symptoms predict declines in physical performance in an elderly, biracial population? *Psychosomatic Medicine* 67:609–15.

26. Penninx, B., et al. (1998). Depressive symptoms and physical decline in community-dwelling older persons. *Journal of American Medical Association* 279(21):1720–6.

27. Callahan, C.M., et al. (1998). Mortality, symptoms and functional impairment in late-life depression. *Journal of General Internal Medicine* 13:746–52.

28. Seeman, T.E., et al. (1995). Behavioral and psychosocial predictors of physical performance: MacArthur Studies of Successful Aging. *Journal of Gerontology: Medical Sciences* 50A(4):M177–83.

29. Fiatarone, M.A., et al. (1994). Exercise training and nutritional supplementation for physical frailty in very elderly people. *New England Journal of Medicine* 330:1769–75.

30. Frontera, W.R., et al. (1988). Strength conditioning in older men: Skeletal muscle hypertrophy and improved function. *Journal of Applied Physiology* 64:1038–44.

31. Pepin, V., Phillips, W.T., Swan, P.D. (2004). Functional assessment of older cardiac rehabilitation patients. *Journal of Cardiopulmonary Rehabilitation* 24:34–7.

32. Black, A.E., et al. (1996). Human energy expenditure in affluent societies: An analysis of 574 doubly-labeled water measurements. *European Journal of Clinical Nutrition* 50:72–92.

33. Westerterp, K.R., Meijer, E.P. (2001). Physical activity and parameters of aging: A physiological perspective. *J Gerontol A Biol Sci Med Sci* 56:7–12.

34. Meijer, E.P., et al. (2001). Physical inactivity as a determinant of the physical activity level in the elderly. *Int J Obes Relat Metab Disord* 25:935–9.

35. Tudor-Locke, C., et al. (2004). Descriptive epidemiology of pedometer-determined physical activity. *Med Sci Sports Exerc* 36(9):1567–73.

36. Petrella, J.K., Cress, M.E. (2004). Daily ambulation activity and task performance in community-dwelling older adults aged 63-71 years with preclinical disability. *J Gerontol A Biol Sci Med Sci* 59:264–7.

37. Hamilton, M.T., Hamilton, D.G., Zderic, T.W. (2004). Exercise physiology versus inactivity physiology: An essential concept for understanding lipoprotein lipase regulation. *Exerc Sport Sci Rev* 32(4):161–6.

38. Zuliani, G., et al. (1997). High-density lipoprotein cholesterol strongly discriminates between healthy free-living and disabled octo-nonagenarians: a cross sectional study. *Aging (Milano)* 9:335–41.

39. Cooper, C., Barker, D.J., Wickham, C. (1988). Physical activity, muscle strength, and calcium intake in fracture of the proximal femur in Britain. *British Medical Journal* 297:1443–6.

40. Feskanich, D., Willett, W., Colditz, G. (2002). Walking and leisure-time activity and risk of hip fracture in postmenopausal women. *The Journal of American Medical Association* 288:2300–6.

41. Weiss, M., Yogev, R., Dolev, E. (1998). Occupational sitting and low hip mineral density. *Calcified Tissue International* 62:47–50.

42. Bertrais, S., et al. (2005). Sedentary behaviors, physical activity, and metabolic syndrome in middle-aged French subjects. *Obesity Research* 13(5):936–44.

43. Dunstan, D.W., et al. (2005) Associations of TV viewing and physical activity with the metabolic syndrome in Australian adults. *Diabetologia* 48(11):2254–61.

44. Ford, E.S., et al. (2005). Sedentary behavior, physical activity, and the metabolic syndrome among U.S. adults. *Obesity Research* 13(3):608–14.

45. Fung, T.T., et al. (2000). Leisure-time physical activity, television watching, and plasma biomarkers of obesity and cardiovascular disease risk. *American Journal of Epidemiology* 152(12):1171–8.

46. Bey, L., et al. (2001). Reduced lipoprotein lipase activity in postural skeletal muscle during aging. *Journal of Applied Physiology* 91(2):687–92.

47. Hamilton, M.T., et al. (2001). Plasma triglyceride metabolism in humans and rats during aging and physical inactivity. *International Journal of Sport Nutrition and Exercise Metabolism* 11(Suppl):S97–104.

48. Bey, L., Hamilton, M.T. (2003). Suppression of skeletal muscle lipoprotein lipase activity during physical inactivity: A molecular reason to maintain daily low-intensity activity. *Journal of Physiology* 551(Pt 2):673–82.

49. Zderic, T.W., Hamilton, M.T. (2006). Physical inactivity amplifies the sensitivity of skeletal muscle to the lipid-induced downregulation of lipoprotein lipase activity. *Journal of Applied Physiology* 100(1):249–57.

50. Coakley, E.H., et al. (1998). Lower levels of physical functioning are associated with higher body weight among middle-aged and older women. *International Journal of Obesity* 22:958–65.

51. Bruce, M.L. (2001). Depression and disability in late life: Directions for future research. *American Journal of Geriatric Psychiatry* 9:102–12.

52. Wang, L., et al. (2002) Predictors of functional change: A longitudinal study of nondemented people aged 65 and older. *Journal of the American Geriatrics Society* 50(9):1525–34.

53. Brach, J.S., et al. (2004). The relationship among physical activity, obesity, and physical function in community-dwelling older women. *Preventive Medicine* 39(1):74–80.

54. Lin, S., Davey, R.C., Cochrane, T. (2004). Community rehabilitation for older adults with osteoarthritis of the lower limb: a controlled clinical trial. *Clinical Rehabilitation* 18(1):92–101.

55. Bellamy, N., Buchanan, W.W., Goldsmith, C.H. (1988). Validation study of the WOMAC: A health status instrument for measuring clinically important patient relevant outcomes to antirheumatic drug therapy in patients with osteoarthritis of the hip or knee. *Journal of Rheumatology* 15:1833–40.

56. Bellamy, N. (1995). Outcome measurement in osteoarthritis clinical trials. *Journal of Rheumatology* 43(Suppl):49–51.

57. American Medical Director's Association. (2003). Pain Management in the Long Term Care Setting: Clinical Practice Guideline. American Medical Directors Association, Columbia, MD.

58. Toraman, F., Sahin, G. (2004). Age responses to multicomponent training program in older adults. *Disability and Rehabilitation* 26(8):448–54.

59. Kenny, A.M., et al. (2003). Effects of vitamin D supplementation on strength, physical function, and health perception in older, community-dwelling men. *Journal of the American Geriatrics* 51(12):1762–7.

60. Rekeneire, N.D., et al. (2003). Is a fall just a fall: Correlates of falling in healthy older persons. The Health, Aging and Body Composition Study. *Journal of the American Geriatrics Society* 51(6):841–6.

61. Podsiadlo, D., Richardson, S. (1991). The timed "Up & Go": A test of basic functional mobility for frail elderly person. *Journal of the American Geriatrics Society* 39:142–8.

62. Reuben, D.B., Siu, A.L. (1990). An objective measure of physical function of elderly outpatients: the physical performance test. *Journal of the American Geriatrics Society* 38:1105–12.

63. Tinetti, M.E. (1986). Performance-oriented assessment of mobility problems in elderly patients. *Journal of the American Geriatrics Society* 34:119–26.

64. Berg, K., et al. (1989). Measuring balance in the elderly: Preliminary development of an instrument. *Physiotherapy Canada* 41(6):304–11.

65. Starner, T.J., et al. (2000). The Gesture Pendant: A self-illuminating, wearable, infrared computer vision system for home automation control and medical monitoring. *Proceedings of IEEE International Symposium on Wearable Computing (ISWC 2000)* Atlanta, GA, October, pp. 87–94.

66. Mihailidis, A., Fernie, G.R., Cleghorn, W.L. (2000). The development of a computerized cueing device to help people with dementia to be more independent. *Technology & Disability* 13(1):23–40.

67. Pollack, M.E., et al. (2003) Autominder: An intelligent cognitive orthotic system for people with memory impairment. *Robotics and Autonomous Systems* 44(3):273–82.

68. Fernie, G., Fernie, B. (1996). The potential role of technology to provide help at home for persons with alzheimer's disease. *Proceedings of the 18th Annual Conference of the Alzheimer's Society of Canada*, Ottawa, ON.

69. Alwan, M., et al. (2003). In-Home Monitoring System and Objective ADL Assessment: Validation Study, International Conference on Independence, Aging and Disability, Washington, DC.

70. Bai, J., et al. (2000). Home telemonitoring framework based on integrated functional modules. *Proceedings of World Congress on Medical Physics and Biomedical Engineering,* Chicago, IL.

71. Nambu, M., et al. (2000). A system to monitor elderly people remotely, using the power line network. *World Congress on Medical Physics and Biomedical Engineering,* Chicago, IL.

72. Dalal S., et al. (2005). A Rule-Based Approach to Analyzing Elders' Activity Data: Detection of Health and Emergency Conditions, Proceedings of the AAAI's Fall Symposium on AI & Eldercare: Caring Machines, Washington, DC, November 2005.

73. Alwan M., et al. (2005).Validation of rule-based inference of selected independent ADLs. *Journal of Telemedicine and E-Health* 11(5):594–9.

74. Mack, D.C., et al. (2006). A passive and portable system for monitoring heart rate and detecting sleep apnea and arousals: Preliminary validation, In *Proceedings of the Transdisciplinary Conference on Distributed Diagnosis and Home Healthcare (D2H2)*, 2–4 April 2006, Arlington, VA.

75. Haigh, K. Z., et al. (2004) The independent lifestyle assistantTM (I.L.S.A.): Deployment lessons learned. *The AAAI 2004 Workshop on Fielding Applications of AI*, 25 July 2004, San Jose, CA, pp. 11–6.

76. Plocher, T., Kiff, L., Krichbaum, K. (2004). Promoting and maximizing independence through new technologies. *AAHSA Future of Aging Services Conference*, 15 March 2004, Washington, DC.

77. Intille, S. (2002). Designing a home of the future. *IEEE Pervasive Computing*, April–June 2002, 80–6.

78. Kidd, C.D., et al. (1999). The aware home: A living laboratory for ubiquitous computing research. In *Proceedings of the Second International Workshop on Cooperative Buildings – CoBuild '99*. October.

79. Mynatt, E.D., et al. (2001). Digital family portraits: Providing peace of mind for extended family members. In *Proceedings of the ACM Conference on Human Factors in Computing Systems (CHI 2001)*. Seattle, WA: ACM Press, pp. 333–40.

80. Bharucha, A., Allin, S., Stevens, S. CareMedia: Towards automated behavior analysis in the nursing home setting. *The International Psychogeriatric Association Eleventh International Congress*, Chicago, IL, 17–22 August 2003.

81. Alwan, M., et al. (2006a). Psychosocial impact of passive health status monitoring technology in assisted living: A pilot study, In *Proceedings of the 2nd IEEE International Conference on Information & Communication Technologies: From Theory to Applications (ICTTA'06)*, 23–28 April 2006, Damascus, Syria.

82. Alwan, M., et al. (2006b). Impact of monitoring technology in assisted living: Outcome pilot. *IEEE Transactions on Information Technology in Medicine and Biology* 10(1):192–8.

83. Alwan, M., et al. (2006d). Impact of passive in-home health status monitoring technology in home health: outcome pilot, In *Proceedings of the Transdisciplinary Conference on Distributed Diagnosis and Home Healthcare (D2H2)*, 2–4 April 2006, Arlington, VA.

84. Alwan M, et al. (2006c). Psychosocial impact of passive health status monitoring on informal caregivers and older adults living in independent senior housing, In *Proceedings of the 2nd IEEE International Conference on Information & Communication Technologies: From Theory to Applications (ICTTA'06)*, 23–28 April 2006, Damascus, Syria.

85. Alwan, M., et al. (2007). Impact of passive health status monitoring to care providers and payers in assisted living. Accepted for publication in *Journal of Telemedicine and E-Health* 13(3):279–286.

86. Barki, H., Hartwick, H.J. (1994). Rethinking the concept of user involvement, and user attitude. *MIS Quarterly* 18(1):59–79.

87. Foster, S.T., Franz, C.R. (1999). User involvement during information systems development: A comparison of analyst and user perceptions of system acceptance. *Journal of Engineering and Technology Management* 16:329–48.

88. Garceau, L., Jancura, E., Kneiss, J. (1993). Object oriented analysis and design: A new approach to systems development. *Journal of Systems Management* 44:25–33.

89. Franz, C.R., Robey, D. (1986). Organisational context, user involvement, and the usefulness of information systems. *Decision Sciences* 17(3):329–56.

90. McKeen, J.D., Guimaraes, T., Wetherbe, J.C. (1994). The relationship between user participation and user satisfaction: An investigation of four contingency factors. *MIS Quarterly* 427–51.

91. Bussen, W.S., Myers, M.D. (1997). Executive information systems failure: a New Zealand case study. PACIS '97, Brisbane, Information systems Management Research Concentration, QUT, Australia.

92. Demiris G., et al. (2006). Nurse participation in the design of user interfaces for a smart home system. 4th International Conference on Smart Homes and Health Telematics Proceedings, Belfast, UK, IOS Press, pp. 66–73.

93. Alexander, G.L., Scott-Cawiezell, J., Wakefield, D.S. (under review). IT sophistication in nursing homes. *Long Term Care Interface.*

94. Telecommunications Industry Association. (1996). Resource guide for accessible design of consumer electronics-linking product design to the needs of people with functional limitations: a joint venture of the electronic industries alliance and the electronic industries foundations. http://www.tiaonline.org/access/guide.html

95. Demiris, G., Finkelstein, S.M., Speedie, S.M. (2001). Considerations for the design of a web-based clinical monitoring and educational system for elderly patients. *JAMIA* 8(5):468–72.

96. Rogers, E. (2003). *Diffusion of Innovations.* 5th ed. New York, The Free Press.

97. Edge, H.M., Milner, J. (1998). Universal design: A social agenda within the ecological designed built environment. Shifting Balance: Changing Roles in Policy, Research and Design, IPAS Conference; 1998; Netherlands.

98. Bopp, K.D., Brown, G.D. (2005). Aligning information strategy and business and clinical strategies: Information as a strategic asset. In Brown, G.D., Stone, T.T., Patrick, T.B. (Eds). *Strategic Management of Information Systems in Healthcare.* Chicago, Health Administration Press, pp. 121–47.

99. Prahalad, C., Ramaswamy, V. (2004). *The Future of Competition.* Boston: Harvard Business School Press, 2004.

100. Ruddick, W. (1994). Transforming homes and hospitals. *The Hastings Center Report* 24(5):s11–4.

101. Abascal, J. (2005). Ambient intelligence for people with disabilities and elderly people. Retrieved 15 October 2005 from http://www.andrew.cmu.edu/course/60-427/aisd/elderly.pdf

102. Hensel, B.K., Demiris, G., Courtney, K.L. (2006). Defining obtrusiveness in home telehealth technologies: A conceptual framework. *Journal of the American Medical Informatics Association* 13(4):428–31.

103. Demiris, G., et al. (in press). Examining senior residents' willingness to adopt smart home sensors. *International Journal of Technology Assessment in Health Care.*

104. Courtney, K.L., Demiris, G., Hensel, B.K. (2007). Obtrusiveness of information-based assistive technologies as perceived by older adults in residential care facilities: A secondary analysis. *Medical Informatics & The Internet in Medicine* 32(3):241–9.

105. Demiris, G., et al. (2004). Older adults' attitudes towards and perceptions of 'smart home' technologies: a pilot study. *Medical Informatics & The Internet in Medicine* 29(2):87–94.

Chapter 3
Mobility and Gait Assessment Technologies

Patrick O. Riley, Kate W. Paylo, and D. Casey Kerrigan

3.1 Introduction

In a past report, the surgeon general implored older adults to engage in regular physical activity (US Department of Health and Human Service, 1999). This same surgeon general report contended that moderate amounts of physical activity, whether short with higher intensity or long with lower intensity, produce significant health benefits. This past insight, coupled with recent improvements in nutrition, medicine, and lifestyle, has led to an increase in the average human lifespan of 30 years since the 1900s [1]. With this increasing segment of the population, developments in gait analysis and exercise physiology have become of paramount importance. The authors attempt to present gait evaluation technology in such a way as to provide the basics for the interpretation of gait cycle analysis. This chapter consists of the terminology and biomechanics of gait, a discussion of the technology used in a clinical gait laboratory, a discussion of office-based technologies for monitoring and assessing mobility, and a description of mobility impairments common among elderly persons.

3.2 Terminology

Considering a single limb, the basic unit of walking and running is one *gait cycle*, or *stride*. At an average walking velocity, the stance period when the foot is in contact with the ground comprises about 60% of the gait cycle, whereas the swing period comprises 40%. Perry and colleagues described eight phases of the gait cycle [2] (Figure 3.1). Events that occur in the gait cycle include *foot contact* (heel strike in heel-toe gait), *foot flat*, *heel rise*, and *foot-off* (toe-off in heel-toe gait). The foot contact event corresponds to the initial contact phase. Foot flat occurs at the end of

Patrick Riley

Research Associate Professor, University of Virginia, School of Medicine, Department of Physical Medicine and Rehabilitation, 545 Ray C. Hunt Drive, Suite 240, Box 801004, Charlottesville, VA 22908-1004
e-mail: por2n@virginia.edu

From: *Aging Medicine, Eldercare Technology for Clinical Practitioners,*
Edited by: M. Alwan and R. Felder © Humana Press, Totowa, NJ

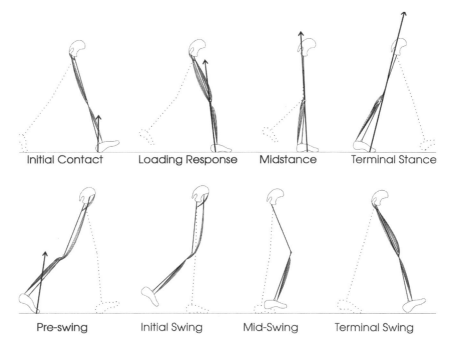

Fig. 3.1 Perry's Eight Gait Phases

the loading response. Heel off begins terminal stance. Foot-off ends pre-swing and begins initial-swing.

Considering both limbs, the gait cycle is divided into two single-support and two double-support periods. Each double-support period lasts from one limb's foot contact to the opposite limb's foot off. Each single-support period corresponds to one limb's swing phase and has duration of approximately 40% of the gait cycle. Thus, about 80% of the gait cycle is spent in single-support, and the two double-support phases are each about 10% of the gait cycle.

Time-distance parameters are used to quantitatively describe gait. *Gait velocity* is simply the speed of gait. *Stride time* is defined from the time of initial contact of one limb with the ground to the next initial contact of the same limb. *Step time* is the duration of time from initial contact of one limb to the time of initial contact of the contra lateral limb. *Stride length* and *step length* refer to the distances covered during their respective times. The *cadence* of gait can be expressed in either strides per minute or steps per minute.

3.3 Gait Biomechanics

Kinematics describes the motions of limb segments and the angular motions of joints. Kinetics describes the moments and forces that cause motion. Similarly, the firing patterns of muscles can be determined with the aid of dynamic electromyography (EMG). The principal advantage of gait laboratory analysis over other forms of gait evaluation is that the gait laboratory measures kinetics, the link between EMG and kinematics.

To appreciate the insight provided by kinetics, it is necessary to consider the biomechanics, the basic physics, of motion. A moment about a joint occurs when a force acts at a distance from the joint. For instance, a weight in the hand produces an externally applied extensor moment about the elbow. In this example, the lever is the forearm and the external moment is the product of the weight of the object and the length of the forearm. The concept of static equilibrium dictates that, in order for the joint angle to remain constant, all the moments acting about the joint must sum to zero. Thus, in our example, for the elbow angle to remain constant, an internal force from the biceps, acting through its muscle lever arm, must provide a resisting internal flexor moment that matches the external extensor moment because of the weight. Small deviations from equilibrium allow stable movement, a condition of dynamic equilibrium. Depending on the magnitude of the biceps force, the elbow joint angle will extend in a controlled fashion (eccentric contraction), stay the same (isometric contraction), or flex (concentric contraction). The controlled accelerations of the body segment masses produce inertial forces, which together with the internal and external moments, sum to zero, a condition of dynamic equilibrium.

During walking, the joints and limb segments are in a state of dynamic equilibrium. The net joint moments match the externally applied forces, including gravity and the body's ground reaction force (GRF), defined as the force exerted by the ground at the point of contact (the feet), and the inertial forces associated with limb segment motion. During the stance period the inertial forces are extremely small; the net joint moments establish equilibrium with the external forces, gravity, and the GRF. During swing, there is no GRF but the inertial forces, although still small, are significant. The joint moments are in equilibrium with the gravitational and inertial forces.

The importance of knowing the direction and magnitude of the GRF and its relationship with muscle behavior and maintenance of equilibrium is best illustrated by the example of quiet standing (Figure 3.2). In quiet standing, the GRF vector extends from the ground through the foot, passing anterior to the ankles and knees, and posterior to the hips. At the hip, passive ligamentous forces transmitted through the iliofemoral ligaments usually are sufficient to counteract the external extensor moment. Similarly, at the knee, the external knee extensor moment is counteracted by the passive forces transmitted through the posterior ligamentous capsule. At the ankle, the external dorsi flexion moment is usually counteracted with an internal ankle plantar flexor moment provided by the ankle plantar flexors. Thus, the only lower extremity muscles that are consistently active during quiet standing are the plantar flexors.

When we walk, the GRF is a function of the position of the body segments and their velocity and acceleration. Knowing where the line of the GRF lies with respect to the hip, knee, and ankle joints gives us a reasonable approximation of the external moments occurring about each of these joints. The GRF can be directly measured with a force plate. Visualizing where the GRF lies with respect to a joint provides

Fig. 3.2 Ground reaction force vector during quiet standing

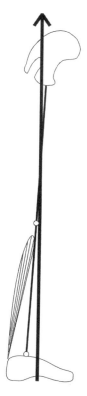

Quiet Standing

a means of approximating the internal moments that must be generated in order to stabilize that joint. For instance, if the GRF line is posterior to the knee, it produces an external knee flexor moment, which is the product of the GRF multiplied by the distance of the GRF line from the axis of the knee joint. To maintain stability so that the knee does not collapse into flexion, an internal knee extensor moment must occur. This moment, provided by the knee extensors, is equal in magnitude to the external flexor moment.

During walking, the GRF vector changes position as the body progresses forward (Figure 3.1). In early-stance, the vector is anterior to the hip and posterior to the knee and ankle. In mid-stance, the vector passes through the hip and knee joints and is anterior to the ankle. During terminal stance, the vector moves posterior to the hip, anterior to the knee joint, and maximally anterior to the ankle. With these dynamics in mind, normal gait function is easier to interpret. The muscles fire in response to the need for joint stability. In quantitative gait analysis, one can determine whether a muscle group is firing concentrically or eccentrically using the joint power, which is mathematically the product of the joint moment and the joint angular velocity.

A positive joint power implies that the muscle group is firing concentrically whereas a negative joint power implies that the muscle group is firing eccentrically.

3.4 Motion Analysis Laboratory Technology

The motion analysis or gait laboratories exist to provide a complete, in-depth, quantitative evaluation of ambulatory function. Gordon Rose, a pioneer in the field, suggested that the term "gait analysis," should be reserved for the high-tech component of gait evaluation performed in the gait laboratory while the more general term "gait assessment" should be applied to the whole process of evaluating a patient's gait [3]. In the diagnostic triad of history, physical examination, and laboratory tests, gait analysis is a laboratory test. Like all laboratory tests, gait analysis should provide answers to specific questions.

A gait laboratory typically uses a combination of three technologies for evaluating the biomechanics of gait.

A motion capture system tracks the patient's movements digitally.
Force plates are used to measure the GRF.
An EMG system is used to record the activity of the muscles in gait.

The information from these components is integrated to provide an understanding of the physiology and mechanics of the patient's gait.

3.4.1 Motion Capture System

The motion capture system, the central and most complex of these technologies, captures a complete description of the gait kinematics in digital form that can then be analyzed and related to other measurements. This process uses the mathematics of photogrammetry; a science that owes its origins to the fields of aerial and satellite mapping. In principle, if one has multiple images of the same object and knows positions, orientations, and optical characteristics of the imaging devices, one can solve for the three-dimensional position of objects from their positions in the two-dimensional pictures.

A state-of-the-art gait laboratory will have a motion capture system consisting of a special purpose computer, interface boxes, and an array of special high-speed video motion capture cameras (motion capture cameras have high sampling frequency of 120 or more frames per second). The motion capture system must be integrated with the force plates and EMG systems. Although the motion capture cameras are based on video technology, they have been tuned for the marker illumination and detection function, and produce no useable video image. The number of cameras will vary depending on the size, configuration, and use of the laboratory; a larger number of cameras do not necessarily indicate a superior laboratory or higher quality data. The laboratory should have a viewing volume sufficient to capture full strides bilaterally. It should also have sufficient space so that the patient is walking at steady state in the viewing volume, not accelerating from the starting position or decelerating to stop just out of the volume.

Although markerless motion capture systems are in development, current practice employs retroreflective or active markers placed on the subject. The motion capture cameras are tuned to image only the markers. To obtain three-dimensional kinematics, each body segment must have at least three markers attached. Segments may share markers at their linking joints, e.g., a knee marker may help define both thigh and shank motion. Typically, fifteen to sixteen markers are used to define lower limb kinematics whereas over thirty markers are required to obtain whole body kinematics. Markers are placed on the body and measurements are taken to define the relationship between the marker locations and the subject's anatomy. A typical set of measurements would include age, height, weight, leg length, and the circumference or diameter of the limbs at various locations. It may also be necessary to use extra markers or a marked pointer to indicate the location of unmarked anatomical landmarks relative to the tracking markers. The marker placement directly affects the quantitative results obtained. Thus, the accuracy and repeatability of motion capture data is dependent on the precision and consistency of marker placement.

3.4.2 Force Plates

Force plates measure the force applied to the ground by the feet as the patient walks over them. They may be thought of as a precision scale, but keep in mind that a force is three-dimensional. The force plates measure not only how hard the person is pushing down on the ground, but also braking and acceleration force, and force directed medio-laterally. This information is integrated with the body kinematics defined by the motion capture system to assess the mechanics of movement.

The number of force plates varies according to the function of the laboratory. At least two plates are required if both limb functions are to be analyzed from a single walk, a desirable but not always achievable goal. If the force plates are not rigidly mounted, they may move when struck or due to floor vibrations producing false signals that can corrupt the biomechanical analysis. This issue arises most frequently in the high-energy dynamics of sports but can manifest its presence in gait analysis.

3.4.3 EMG

The EMG system is used to record the activity of muscles during gait, a process referred to as dynamic EMG. EMG is generally recorded using either passive or active surface electrodes. Active electrodes are rigid and have a built-in amplifier.

They are less susceptible to artifacts because of wire motion but are more susceptible to artifacts because of electrode motion relative to the skin. EMG electrodes may be interfaced with the data collection system through an umbilical cable or with a telemetric system using a small radio transmitter and power pack. The EMG system will typically be set up to monitor a number of muscles simultaneously.

Surface electrodes cannot readily be used to detect the activity of deep muscles, e.g., the tibialis posterior. In addition, surface EMG is subject to cross talk, particularly when a rather small muscle is adjacent to larger muscles with overlapping firing patterns, e.g., the rectus femoris. If the EMG of such muscles is required, fine wire electrodes are used. Proper electrode placement and the absence of cross talk in the fine wire electrodes should be verified by electronic muscle stimulation. Although the process is relatively safe and effective, the procedure adds significantly to the complexity of gait analysis. Physicians desiring fine wire EMG should specifically request it in their referral and indicate the reason for so requesting.

Analysis of EMG can be done on several levels. The most basic level is asking whether the activity of a muscle is phasic or is nearly constant. The next level of analysis asks whether the muscle activity occurs at the normal time in the gait cycle. Examining only the timing of muscle activity assumes that the patient's gait is normal, in which case they should not be undergoing gait analysis. If the patient's posture or movement dynamics are abnormal, it follows that the mechanics of movement are altered; hence, the activity of the muscle driving their movement will also be altered. EMG analysis should first assess whether the muscle activity is appropriate to produce the forces acting at that instant to produce the existing gait pattern, and second, ask whether the manifest forces are contributing to or inhibiting the desired movement. Muscle activity can only be effectively assessed from the logical interpretation of these two questions; i.e., it can only be assessed in conjunction with the kinematics and kinetics of gait. Hence, the closest possible coupling between EMG and motion capture and force plate data is desirable.

3.4.4 Metabolic Function

Given the increasing prevalence of medical co-morbidities in the aging population, the energy cost of walking is an extremely important factor. The amount of energy consumed while walking can be determined using indirect calorimetry, i.e., by measuring the patient's oxygen consumption and carbon dioxide production. The ratio of carbon dioxide production to oxygen consumption also indicates whether the patient has exceeded their anaerobic threshold. There is ample evidence that patients adjust their gait to avoid exceeding their maximum aerobic capacity (VO_2 max). These measurements can be used to determine whether the patient may benefit from conditioning or whether an intervention improves gait efficiency.

Historically, these measurements were made by collecting exhaled gasses over a period. Recently, instrumentation has become available to measure these parameters on a breath-by-breath basis. This instrumentation is more compact, portable and comfortable than the older equipment. To determine the metabolic cost of walking, it is necessary to subtract the average resting oxygen consumption from the average obtained during steady-state ambulation. Walking at constant speed on a clear track or treadmill for several minutes is required for the latter measurement. These requirements are not consistent with normal motion capture procedures and metabolic measurements are usually made independently of gait analysis trials. The results are affected by the patient's level of fatigue, recent diet, and general condition.

3.4.5 Treadmills

Treadmills can be used to allow gait to be observed for prolonged periods of time. Kinematics may be obtained if the treadmill is positioned in the motion capture system viewing volume. Treadmills with instrumentation to measure the vertical component of the GRF are commercially available. Recently, treadmill force plates have been developed, which may permit analysis of both the kinematics and the kinetics of treadmill gait.

3.4.6 Foot Pressure Analysis

Force plates measure the total force because of the foot contacting the ground but do not measure how the load is distributed over the plantar surface of the foot. This information is of interest in dealing with patients with neuropathies and in defining the extent of and risks associated with foot deformities.

Two technologies are used to measure the plantar surface load distribution. The first is a floor-mounted device similar in appearance to a force plate but divided into many small regions. The vertical force applied to each region is measured and used to calculate the pressure on the portion of the plantar surface above that region. As with a force plate, the measurement is made only when the foot is on the plate. These systems have high resolution, and their results are quite repeatable.

The second technology uses flexible inserts between the foot and the shoe. The insert is again subdivided into a number of regions, and each region is instrumented to measure the local force. The resolution of these devices is generally lower than that of the fixed plates. The measurements are affected by how the foot, shoe, and insert fit, and the load sensors tend to be less precise and less uniform than those used in the floor-mounted platforms. However, measurements for a number of steps may be obtained, and orthotics may be evaluated under conditions of actual use. Both technologies were developed as adjuncts to gait laboratory testing but may be used independently in the clinic or care facility.

3.4.7 Normal Kinematic and Kinetic Parameters

The following descriptions of normal sagittal plane kinematics and kinetics are based on data collected from the Spaulding Rehabilitation Hospital Gait Laboratory (Figure 3.3) and are similar to those reported elsewhere. The general patterns of movement are representative of adults and non-disabled children older than 3 years of age [4]. Figure 3.1 illustrates the chief actions occurring in each phase with a visual representation of the limb and joint positions, the GRF line, and the muscles that are active during that phase.

3.4.8 Initial Contact

Initial contact with the ground typically occurs with the heel. The hip is flexed at 30°, the knee is almost fully extended, and the ankle is in a neutral position. As the GRF is anterior to the hip, the hip extensors (gluteus maximus and hamstrings) are firing to maintain hip stability. At the knee, the GRF creates an external extensor moment, which is counteracted by hamstring activity. The foot is supported in the neutral position by the ankle dorsi flexors.

3.4.9 Loading Response

During this phase, weight acceptance and shock absorption are achieved while maintaining forward progression. The hip extends and will continue to extend into the terminal stance phase. The GRF is anterior to the hip, and the hip extensors must be active to resist uncontrolled hip flexion. Active hip extension implies that the hip extensors are concentrically active. With the location of the GRF now posterior to the knee joint, an external flexor moment is created. This external moment is resisted by an eccentric contraction of the quadriceps allowing knee flexion to approximately 20°. With the GRF posterior to the ankle, an external plantar flexion moment occurs that rapidly lowers the foot into 10° of plantar flexion. This action is controlled by the ankle dorsi flexors, which fire eccentrically. At the end of loading response, the foot is in full contact with the ground.

3.4.10 Mid-Stance

During mid-stance, the limb supports the full body weight as the contra lateral limb swings forward. The GRF vector passes through the hip joint, eliminating the need for hip extensor activity. At the knee, the GRF moves from a posterior to an anterior position, similarly eliminating the need for quadriceps activity. Knee extension occurs and is restrained passively by the knee's posterior ligamentous capsule, and is

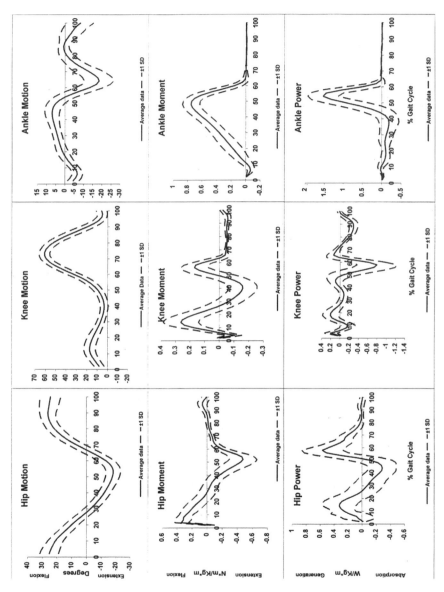

Fig. 3.3 Normal sagittal plane kinematics and kinetics data (based on the Spaulding Rehabilitation Hospital Gait Laboratory)

possibly actively restrained as well by eccentric popliteus and gastrocnemius action. At the ankle, the GRF is anterior to the ankle, thus producing an external ankle dorsi flexion moment. This moment is counteracted by the ankle planar flexors, which eccentrically limit the dorsi flexion occurring during this phase.

3.4.11 Terminal Stance

In terminal stance, the body's mass continues to progress over the limb as the trunk falls forward. The GRF at the hip is now posterior, creating an extensor moment countered passively by the iliofemoral ligaments. The hip is maximally extended. At the knee, the GRF moves from an anterior to a posterior position. As the heel rises from the ground, the GRF moves further anterior to the ankle joint generating an external dorsi flexion moment that is balanced by ankle planar flexor activity. During this phase, the ankle is planar flexing, and thus the action of the ankle planar flexors has switched from eccentric to concentric.

3.4.12 Pre-Swing

During pre-swing, the limb begins to be propelled forward into swing. This phase is occurring as the contra lateral limb advances through initial contact and loading response. From maximal hip extension, the hip begins flexing because of the combined activation of the iliopsoas, hip adductors, and rectus femoris, which are concentrically active. The knee quickly flexes to $40°$ as the GRF progresses rapidly posterior to the knee. Knee flexion may be controlled by rectus femoris activity. The ankle planar flexes to approximately $20°$ because of continued concentric activity of the ankle planar flexors.

3.4.13 Initial Swing

During initial swing, the limb is propelled forward. Hip flexion occurs because of the hip flexion momentum initiated in pre-swing and because of continued concentric activity of the hip flexors. The rectus femoris and vastus lateralis work independently during initial swing phase, with the rectus femoris activity directly correlated to walking speed [5]. The rectus femoris is active during both loading response and pre- and initial-swing phases, regardless of walking speed, with much variability in patterns of muscular activity. Some subjects exhibit greater activity during late stance, whereas others have higher EMG amplitudes during early stance [6]. The knee continues to flex to approximately $65°$. Knee flexion occurs passively as a combined result of hip flexion and the momentum generated from pre-swing. The ankle dorsi flexors are concentrically dorsi flexing the ankle to provide toe clearance.

3.4.14 Mid-Swing

In mid-swing, the limb continues to advance forward, primarily passively as a pendulum, from inertial forces generated in pre- and initial swing. The momentum generated in initial swing passively flexes the hip. The knee begins to extend passively because of gravity. The ankle remains in a neutral position with the continued activity of the ankle dorsi flexors.

3.4.15 Terminal Swing

In terminal swing, the previously generated momentum is controlled to provide stable limb alignment at initial contact. At the hip and knee joints, strong eccentric contraction of the hamstrings decelerates hip flexion and controls knee extension. The ankle dorsi flexors remain active allowing a neutral ankle position at initial contact.

3.4.16 Coronal Plane Motion

Although lower extremity motion during gait occurs primarily in the sagittal plane, coronal plane motion is also of clinical interest. At initial contact, the pelvis and hip are in neutral positions in the coronal plane. During much of the stance period, the GRF passes medial to the hip, knee, and ankle joint centers as the opposite limb is unloading. This medial GRF about the hip causes an external adductor moment that allows the contralateral side of the pelvis to drop slightly. This motion is controlled by eccentric contraction of the hip abductors. During stance, the GRF position medial to the knee imposes an external varus moment about the knee, which must be counteracted by lateral ligament and tendon tension, eccentric muscle activity, and compression forces to the medial compartment of the knee. The presence of a varus moment throughout most of stance contributes to osteoarthritis of the knee, which most typically occurs in the medial compartment of the knee. The varus moment can be affected by external biomechanical factors such as shoewear [7].

3.5 Mobility Assessment Technology Outside the Gait Laboratory

Motion analysis laboratories are large, complex, and expensive facilities. The number of clinical motion analysis laboratories has increased, but availability is still limited. The cost of a full gait evaluation is not justified for routine mobility assessment. Furthermore, the motion laboratory walkway is not representative of the complex environment within which an elderly person must function. The clinical motion analysis community is seeking to address these limitations.

There is also a perceived need to develop mobility analysis technologies that can be used in the clinician's office, the patient's home or care facility, or the community. Such technology can be used as a diagnostic or screening tool, to assess function and determine whether an intervention is warranted or to determine whether an ongoing intervention is effective. These technologies can provide objective quantitative measures to document the efficacy of a treatment protocol, a function that will become increasingly important as health care resources become more strained and health care providers are held more accountable.

3.5.1 Video Recording

Video recordings are used to augment observational gait analysis and provide a degree of quality control for the motion capture data. In the gait laboratory, the subject is viewed from one side and the front/back using at least two cameras. Additional cameras may be used to view the subject from above or from both sides simultaneously, which can be helpful in understanding the subject's movement patterns. All cameras are synchronized and the views are integrated into a single image. Slow motion and even frame-by-frame playback may be used as an adjunct to observational gait analysis, enabling quick or subtle movements to be more readily detected.

Video recordings can be used to document the patient's mobility function and how it changes over time. Slow motion and repeated play can be used to augment visual observation. Patients can be shown specific features of their movement pattern and how recommended modifications will improve their mobility. Using digital video recording cameras operating at higher sampling frequency than regular video cameras (60 fames per second as opposed to 30 frames per second for standard NTSC video cameras) and user-friendly video editing and CD/DVD-recording software, the patient can be given an annotated recording of their evaluation. Using appropriate software and procedures, basic measurement scan can be made using this technology. The athletic coaching and sports medicine communities have been the primary users of this technology (e.g., http//www.sports-motion.com/introduction.htm), but it has potential application to all forms of mobility assessment.

3.5.2 Gait Mats and Stride Analyzers

Devices can be used to record foot placement or the timing of several steps. Gait mats are used to record foot placement over several steps. These devices allow direct measurement of distance parameters, e.g., stride length and step width. Combined with a stopwatch or infrared detectors to determine mat transit time, the temporal distance parameters of gait, cadence and velocity, can be measured. Because several strides can be recorded, some measures of the variability of these parameters can be obtained. The earliest form of gait mat was a wide role of carbon paper. Each step left a trace on the paper from which measurements could be obtained. Modern mats employ technology similar to that used to record foot pressure distribution. The mat sensors are larger than the pressure sensors, providing less special resolution. They are generally not calibrated to produce pressure measurements, but only to determine whether a pressure threshold has been exceeded, indicating when and where contact has occurred. Measurements obtained from these devices have been validated [8–11]. For example, for slow gait, average measurements from the GAITRite® gait mat and the Vicon® motion capture system agreed to within 2.4 cm (3.4%) for stride length, 0.03 s (5.9%) for step time, and 0.02 m/s (1.4%) for gait speed [12]. Gait mats are widely used in clinical research [13–36].

Wearable footswitch-based stride analyzers were originally developed as an adjunct technology for gait laboratories. Functioning independently, they are capable of measuring the timing of gait cycle events and the variability of these parameters. Distance parameters can be estimated if strides are recorded over a measured distance. The repeatability of time distance parameters has been documented [37]. Both its clinical use as a screening tool [38] and its use in research to provide objective quantitative measure of gait characteristics [39, 40] have been documented.

3.5.3 Wearable Monitors

Accelerometers and gyroscopes have been used to detect gait cycle events and monitor activity. Accelerometers detect the inertial forces acting on a mass as it is moved through space. Gyroscopes sense the forces acting on an inertial mass because of a change in orientation in space. Thus, accelerometers sense changes in linear motion, whereas gyroscopes sense changes in orientation. If these devices are firmly attached to a body segment, they will undergo the same linear and angular motion as that body segment. The motion patterns of a body segment repeat with some degree of variability each gait cycle. Certain features of the pattern correspond to gait cycle events. By detecting the repeating pattern and features within the pattern, accelerometers and gyroscopes can track gait cycles and record the timing of gait cycle events. With a bit more processing, the sensor output can also be used to detect non-cyclic events: turns, stair assents, sitting in and rising from a chair; the various activities of daily living.

Modern accelerometer and gyroscope packages are small with dimensions in the order of millimeters and masses of a few grams. Processing and recording the data and providing power require a package not much larger than a cell phone. Thus, these devices can conceivably be used for long-term community activity monitoring; serving as a Holter Monitor for ambulation. A commercially available accelerometer-based device, the intelligent device for energy expenditure and activity (IDEEA) recorder, was shown to correctly identify posture and limb movements with an accuracy of 98.9% and gait types with an accuracy of 98.5% under laboratory conditions [41]. Studies have also validated the gait classification ability of gyroscope-based devices [42, 43].

3.5.4 Environmental Monitors

Because ambulation results in GRFs, it produces a detectable effect on the environment. Anyone who has listened to someone descending wooden steps or walking in the room above them knows that the foot–floor interaction contains a great deal of information about gait, frequently sufficient to identify the walker. Accelerometers, strain gages, and similar devices attached to the floor or supporting structures, can detect these unique signatures. Using pattern recognition and feature extraction algorithms similar to those employed with the wearable technologies described above, information about the walker's gait and activity level can be derived.

This technology is, of course, not portable. By activating sensors in the office or therapy gym floor, the technology can be used to obtain objective, quantitative data as an adjunct to observational gait evaluation [44]. Built-in sensors can be used to perform monitoring functions in residential care facilities. The University of Virginia Medical Automation Research Center's Smarthouse incorporates such technology to monitor activity and detect falls (http://marc.med.virginia.edu/projects_smarthomemonitor.html). The technology is relatively inexpensive and unobtrusive. In addition to dealing with the technical issues of environmental noise and interference from other ambulators, there are also legal and psychosocial issues related to unobtrusive, but constant, monitoring of activity. Such privacy issues can be overcome with adequate safeguards and more than offset by the benefits of prolonging independent living.

3.5.5 Instrumented Walking Aids

The next chapter will describe intelligent aids to ambulation. These devices use sensors and artificial intelligence to sense the user's intent, to anticipate his or her requirements. This technology almost implicitly provides these devices with the ability to monitor the user's mobility [45]. These technologies, as the environmental monitoring technologies described previously, are in a relatively early stage of development. However, they hold significant promise for the near future as a component of telemedicine-supported geriatric medicine.

3.6 Atypical Gait Patterns Associated with Aging

Gait analysis is extremely useful when characterizing gait pattern alterations associated with aging. There have been three principle foci of investigation leading to elder gait pathologies: alterations because of reduced strength, alterations because of impaired balance control, and alterations because of limited range of motion. Although subtle differences have been identified in the gait patterns of elders as a group compared with that of healthy young persons, there is no well-defined elder gait pattern [46, 47].

3.6.1 Atypical Gait Patterns Associated with Weak Ankle Dorsi Flexors

Dorsi flexor weakness has a characteristic gait pattern that may be observed in patients with peroneal nerve palsy. This occurs because of nerve entrapment at the fibular head or more proximally as an injury to a branch of the sciatic nerve. It may also occur in an L-5 radiculopathy. If the ankle dorsi flexors have a motor strength grade of 3/5 or 4/5, the characteristic clinical sign is "foot slap" occurring after initial contact, because of the inability of the ankle dorsi flexors to eccentrically contract to control the rate of plantar flexion after heel contact. If the ankle dorsi flexors have a motor strength grade less than 3/5, toe drag and/or a steppage gait pattern with excessive hip flexion in swing will occur. The cause of these patterns can usually be determined with a careful history, physical examination, and standard electrodiagnostic procedures.

3.6.2 Gait Patterns Associated with Impaired Strength and/or Power-Generating Capacity

It is widely documented that elderly persons tend to walk more slowly with reduced step length. Reduced step length may be due to impaired balance or fear of falling. However, gait analysis kinetic parameters have been examined to determine whether reduced speed is the result of reduced strength or agility. The role of strength may be assessed by examining the maximum net moment developed at each joint in gait. The role of agility may be assessed by examining the maximum power generated at each joint. Judge et al. [48] and Riley et al. [49] found that elders, when asked to walk fast, did not increase their maximum ankle plantar flexor moment. This implies that impaired push-off may be a factor limiting gait speed although linear power-flow analyses indicate that there is not a direct link between push-off and propulsion [50, 51]. Kerrigan et al., in a study of a larger group, found that healthy elderly subjects were able to increase their peak ankle plantar flexor moment and power in order to walk faster. There is evidence that lower extremity strength improves mobility and gait speed [52].

3.6.3 Gait Patterns Associated with Impaired Balance Control

Although strength affects balance control [53], a number of other functions with known age-associated changes are also factors. Vision and somatosensory function commonly deteriorate with age, particularly in the presence of diabetes and peripheral vascular disease. The vestibular system may also be impaired with age secondary to otolith degradation and subtle changes in cerebellar function. These age-related changes can impair gait and mobility [54]. Chapter 8 will address balance and fall risk assessment as well as fall detection and prevention technologies.

3.6.4 Alterations in Gait Because of Restricted Range of Motion and Flexibility

The mobility of elders may also be adversely affected by the loss of flexibility and range of motion. In particular, Kerrigan et al. found that maximum hip extension was restricted in healthy elders compared with that in young persons [55] and even more restricted in elders who tend to fall [56]. Furthermore, exercise programs that specifically increase hip extension range of motion improve gait speed and normalize pelvic kinematics [57]. Gait analysis is extremely effective in determining the dynamic hip range of motion compared with classic methods such as the Thomas Test [58]. These findings suggest that assessment of flexibility is important in elderly patients and that dynamic measures such as gait analysis may be more sensitive and specific than the classic physical examination.

References

1. Santrock, J.W. *Life-Span development* 2002, New York: McGraw Hill.
2. Perry, J. *Gait Analysis: normal and pathological function* 1992, Thorofare: SLACK, Inc.
3. Rose, G.K. Clinical gait assessment: a personal view. *Journal of Medical Engineering & Technology* 1983, **7**(6): p. 273–9.
4. Sutherland, D.H., et al. *The Development of Mature Walking* 1988, Philadelphia: Mac Keith Press.
5. Nene, A., R. Mayagoitia, and P. Veltink. Assessment of rectus femoris function during initial swing phase. *Gait & Posture* 1999, **9**(1): p. 1–9.
6. Annaswamy, T.M., et al. Rectus femoris: Its role in normal gait. *Archives of Physical Medicine & Rehabilitation* 1999, **80**: p. 930–4.
7. Kerrigan, D., M. Todd, and P. Riley. Knee osteoarthritis and high-heeled shoes. *Lancet* 1998, **351**(9113): p. 1399–401.
8. Bilney, B., M. Morris, and K. Webster. Concurrent related validity of the GAITRite walkway system for quantification of the spatial and temporal parameters of gait. *Gait & Posture* 2003, **17**(1): p. 68–74.
9. Nelson, A.J., et al. The validity of the GaitRite and the functional ambulation performance scoring system in the analysis of Parkinson gait. *NeuroRehabilitation* 2002, **17**(3): p. 255–62.
10. McDonough, A.L., et al. The validity and reliability of the GAITRite system's measurements: A preliminary evaluation. *Arch Phys Med Rehabil* 2001, **82**(3): p. 419–25.
11. Cutlip, R.G., et al. Evaluation of an instrumented walkway for measurement of the kinematic parameters of gait. *Gait & Posture* 2000, **12**(2): p. 134–8.
12. Morris, M.E., et al. Short-term relationships between footstep variables in young adults. *Gait & Posture* 2006, 229–35
13. Webster, K.E., J.E. Wittwer, and J.A. Feller. Validity of the GAITRite walkway system for the measurement of averaged and individual step parameters of gait. *Gait & Posture* 2005, **22**(4): p. 317–21.
14. Dusing, S.C. and D.E. Thorpe. A normative sample of temporal and spatial gait parameters in children using the GAITRite((R)) electronic walkway. *Gait & Posture* 2006, 135–9.
15. Chien, S.L., et al. The efficacy of quantitative gait analysis by the GAITRite system in evaluation of parkinsonian bradykinesia. *Parkinsonism & Related Disorders* 2006, 438–42.
16. Camicioli, R., T. Bouchard, and L. Licis. Dual-tasks and walking fast: Relationship to extrapyramidal signs in advanced Alzheimer disease. *Journal of Neurological Sciences* 2006.

17. Guzian, M.C., et al. Orthopaedic shoes improve gait in a Charcot-Marie-Tooth patient: a combined clinical and quantified case study. *Prosthetics and Orthotics International* 2006, **30**(1): p. 87–96.

18. Kressig, R.W. and O. Beauchet. Guidelines for clinical applications of spatio-temporal gait analysis in older adults. *Aging Clinical & Experimental Research* 2006, **18**(2): p. 174–6.

19. Yang, Y.R., et al. Dual-task-related gait changes in individuals with stroke. *Gait & Posture* 2007, **25**(2): p. 185–90.

20. Lin, P.Y., et al. The relation between ankle impairments and gait velocity and symmetry in people with stroke. *Archives of Physical Medicine and Rehabilitation* 2006, **87**(4): p. 562–8.

21. Toole, T., et al. The effects of loading and unloading treadmill walking on balance, gait, fall risk, and daily function in Parkinsonism. *NeuroRehabilitation* 2005, **20**(4): p. 307–22.

22. Thorpe, D.E., S.C. Dusing, and C.G. Moore. Repeatability of temporospatial gait measures in children using the GAITRite electronic walkway. *Archives of Physical Medicine and Rehabilitation* 2005, **86**(12): p. 2342–6.

23. Shore, W.S., et al. A comparison of gait assessment methods: Tinetti and GAITRite electronic walkway. *Journal of the American Geriatrics Society* 2005, **53**(11): p. 2044–5.

24. Chamberlin, M.E., et al. Does fear of falling influence spatial and temporal gait parameters in elderly persons beyond changes associated with normal aging? *The Journals of Gerontology. Series A, Biological Sciences and Medical Sciences* 2005, **60**(9): p. 1163–7.

25. Ng, S.S. and C.W. Hui-Chan. The timed up & go test: its reliability and association with lower-limb impairments and locomotor capacities in people with chronic stroke. *Archives of Physical Medicine and Rehabilitation* 2005, **86**(8): p. 1641–7.

26. Menz, H.B., et al. Response to Letter to the Editor: Reliability of the GAITRite((R)) walkway system for the quantification of temporo-spatial parameters of gait in young and older people. *Gait & Posture* 2006, **23**(4): p. 524–5.

27. Parmar, V., A.J. Shyam Kumar, and W.M. Harper. Reliability of the GAITRite walkway system for the quantification of temporo-spatial parameters of gait in young and older people. *Gait & Posture* 2006, **23**(4): p. 523; author reply 524–5.

28. Almeida, Q.J., et al. An evaluation of sensorimotor integration during locomotion toward a target in Parkinson's disease. *Neuroscience* 2005, **134**(1): p. 283–93.

29. Rao, A.K., L. Quinn, and K.S. Marder. Reliability of spatiotemporal gait outcome measures in Huntington's disease. *Movement Disorders* 2005, **20**(8): p. 1033–7.

30. Camicioli, R. and L. Licis. Motor impairment predicts falls in specialized Alzheimer care units. *Alzheimer Disease and Associated Disorders* 2004, **18**(4): p. 214–8.

31. Menz, H.B., et al. Reliability of the GAITRite walkway system for the quantification of temporo-spatial parameters of gait in young and older people. *Gait & Posture* 2004, **20**(1): p. 20–5.

32. van Uden, C.J. and M.P. Besser. Test-retest reliability of temporal and spatial gait characteristics measured with an instrumented walkway system (GAITRite). *BMC Musculoskeletal Disorders* 2004, **5**: p. 13.

33. Titianova, E.B., P.S. Mateev, and I.M. Tarkka. Footprint analysis of gait using a pressure sensor system. *Journal of Electromyography and Kinesiology* 2004, **14**(2): p. 275–81.

34. Patla, A.E., T.C. Davies, and E. Niechwiej. Obstacle avoidance during locomotion using haptic information in normally sighted humans. *Experimental Brain Research* 2004, **155**(2): p. 173–85.

35. Thomas, M., et al. Clinical gait and balance scale (GABS): Validation and utilization. *Journal of Neurological Sciences* 2004, **217**(1): p. 89–99.

36. Silverberg, R., et al. Gait variables of patients after lower extremity burn injuries. *The Journal of Burn Care and Rehabilitation* 2000, **21**(3): p. 259–67; discussion 258.

37. Hill, K.D., et al. Retest reliability of the temporal and distance characteristics of hemiplegic gait using a footswitch system. *Archives of Physical Medicine and Rehabilitation* 1994, **75**: p. 577–83.

38. Harada, N., et al. Screening for balance and mobility impairment in elderly individuals living in residential care facilities. *Physical Therapy* 1995, **75**(6): p. 462–9.

39. Peterson, M.G., et al. Effect of a walking program on gait characteristics in patients with osteoarthritis. *Arthritis Care and Research* 1993, **6**(1): p. 11–6.
40. Powers, C.M., et al. Stair ambulation in persons with transtibial amputation: an analysis of the Seattle LightFoot. *Journal of Rehabilitation Research and Development* 1997, **34**(1): p. 9–18.
41. Zhang, K., et al. Measurement of human daily physical activity. *Obesity Research* 2003, **11**: p. 33–40.
42. Miyazaki, S. Long-term unrestrained measurement of stride length and walking velocity utilizing a piezoelectric gyroscope. *IEEE Transactions on Biomedical Engineering* 1997, **44**(8): p. 753–9.
43. Tong, K. and M.H. Granat. A practical gait analysis system using gyroscopes. *Medical Engineering & Physics* 1999, **21**(2): p. 87–94.
44. Alwan, M., et al. Derivation of Basic Human Gait Characteristics From Floor Vibrations. In Summer Bioengineering Conference, 2003, Key Biscayne, Florida.
45. Alwan, M., et al. Passive Derivation of Basic Walker-Assisted Gait Characteristics from Measured Forces and Moments in EMBC. 2004.
46. Imms, F.J. and O.G. Edholm. Studies of gait and mobility in the elderly. *Age and Aging* 1981, **10**: p. 147–156.
47. Winter, D.A., A.E. Patla, J.S. Frank, and S.E. Walt. Biomechanical walking pattern changes in the fit and healthy elderly. *Physical Therapy* 1990, **70**: p. 340–347.
48. Judge, J.O., R.B. Davis, 3rd, and S. Ounpuu. Step length reductions in advanced age: the role of ankle and hip kinetics. *The Journals of Gerontology. Series A, Biological Sciences and Medical Sciences* 1996, **51**(6): p. M303–12.
49. Riley, P.O., U. DellaCroce, and D.C. Kerrigan. Effect of age on lower extremity joint moment contributions to gait speed. *Gait & Posture* 2001, **14**(3): p. 264–70.
50. Meinders, M., A. Gitter, and J.M. Czerniecki. The role of ankle plantar flexor muscle work during walking. *Scandinavian Journal of Rehabilitation Medicine* 1998, **30**(1): p. 39–46.
51. Riley, P.O., U. Della Croce, and D.C. Kerrigan. Propulsive adaptation to changing gait speed. *Journal of Biomechanics* 2001, **34**(2): p. 197–202.
52. Chandler, J.M., et al. Is lower extremity strength gain associated with improvement in physical performance and disability in frail, community-dwelling elders? *Archives of Physical Medicine and Rehabilitation* 1998, **79**(1): p. 24–30.
53. Kerrigan, D.C., et al. Kinetic alterations independent of walking speed in elderly fallers. *Archives of Physical Medicine and Rehabilitation* 2000, **81**(6): p. 730–5.
54. Duncan, P.W., et al. How do physiological components of balance affect mobility in elderly men? *Archives of Physical Medicine and Rehabilitation* 1993, **74**(12): p. 1343–9.
55. Kerrigan, D.C., et al. Biomechanical gait alterations independent of speed in the healthy elderly: Evidence for specific limiting impairments. *Archives of Physical Medicine and Rehabilitation* 1998, **79**(3): p. 317–22.
56. Kerrigan, D., et al. Reduced hip extension during walking: healthy elderly and fallers versus young adults. *Archives of Physical Medicine and Rehabilitation* 2001, **82**: p. 26–30.
57. Kerrigan, D.C., et al. Effect of a hip flexor stretching program on gait in the elderly. *Archives of Physical Medicine and Rehabilitation* 2003, **84**: p. 1–6.
58. Lee, L.W., D.C. Kerrigan, and U. Della Croce. Dynamic implications of hip flexion contractures. *American Journal of Physical Medicine and Rehabilitation* 1997, **76**(6): p. 502–8.

Chapter 4
Intelligent Mobility Aids for the Elderly

Glenn Wasson, Pradip Sheth, Cunjun Huang, and Majd Alwan

4.1 Introduction

One of the most important factors in quality of life for older adults is their ability to move about independently. Not only is mobility crucial for performing the activities of daily living (ADLs) and instrumental activities of daily living (IADLs), for example, shopping, but also for maintaining fitness and vitality. Lack of independence and exercise can lead to a vicious cycle. Decreased mobility because of a perceived lack of safety can cause muscular atrophy and a loss of the feeling of empowerment (both of which contribute to further decreased mobility). Mobility is not only important for vitality of the individual but for the health of the community as well. Older adults often have a significant stake in their local community and can be motivated contributors to its well-being. Even participation in the community at the level of instrumented ADLs, such as shopping and using public transportation, requires a degree of personal mobility, and these IADLs are among the first to be lost by older adults [1].

Intelligent mobility aids for the elderly represent a new class of assistive devices that attempt to augment the user's current abilities instead of replacing them. Although intelligent wheelchairs have a rich history [2–7], other mobility aids such as the cane and the walker are used by more than four times as many people as those who use wheelchairs, totaling some 6.5 million people [8]. Intelligent versions of these aids have, until recently, received much less attention. However, recent advances have created mobility aids that can provide judicious assistance in difficult or dangerous situations while remaining quiescent otherwise. By assessing their user's intent through natural means, that is, without explicit direction from the user, these aids can work collaboratively with their users without an increase in the user's cognitive load. In other words, these aids seek to provide the benefits of mobility and exercise with increased safety while simultaneously providing the same "feel" as their traditional, non-intelligent, non-computer-controlled counterparts.

Glenn Wasson
Dept. of Computer Science, University of Virginia
e-mail: wasson@virginia.edu

From: *Aging Medicine, Eldercare Technology for Clinical Practitioners,*
Edited by: M. Alwan and R. Felder © Humana Press, Totowa, NJ

There are also significant economic reasons for pursuing mobility aid technology. In 1997, there were over 68 million people with activity limitations in the USA [9]. Limitations in activity increase with age and among those 65–74 years old, 26.1% reported a limitation caused by a chronic condition in the year 2000. In contrast, almost half (45.1%) of those 75 years and over reported they were limited by chronic conditions. The percentage of individuals with disabilities increases sharply with age. Disability takes a much heavier toll on the very old. Almost three-quarters (73.6%) of those aged 80+ report at least one disability. Over half (57.6%) of those aged 80+ had one or more severe disabilities and 34.9% of the 80+ population reported needing assistance as a result of disability. Arthritis alone affected 40% of older adults over the age of 65 [10]. Moreover, the world's elderly population is rising. In the USA, the elderly population is expected to double over the next 30 years [11]. In Japan, already the country with the highest percentage of citizens over the age of 65, one in four people will be over 65 by 2030. That same age bracket will reach 17% of the global population by 2050 [12]. At the same time, healthcare costs in the USA are expected to increase to $4 trillion [13], and the oldest 10% of the US population already accounts for more than 50% of healthcare expenses [14]. Direct medical costs from fall-related injuries (one of the primary risks mitigated by mobility aids) total over $19 billion annually [15].

This chapter addresses two inter-related issues in intelligent mobility aids: how to determine what the user is doing (or where they want to go) and how to activate appropriate control to help them attain their goal. The first issue is partly a user-interface problem, how to extract information from the user, and partly a question of interpreting that information (i.e., deriving "meaning" from the input or finding the "signal" in the noise). We discuss the use of natural, force-based input and the interpretation of such signals. The second issue deals with designing a control system that respects the fact that the walker system is actually a multi-body system in which both the user and the walker frame are affected by the walker frame's motion. In such systems, control must be designed not to maximize travel speed or clearance but user safety and stability. In other words, in some situations, it may be reasonable to impact an object rather than make a destabilizing movement to avoid it. We discuss the use of passive, shared control in a control system that dynamically shifts the degree of control between the walker and the human depending on the circumstances and the immediate environment.

The remainder of this chapter is organized as follows. Section 4.2 discusses related work in the field of mobility aids, both using walkers and other devices. Section 4.3 describes a philosophy and overall architecture for assessing user intent and implementing passive, shared control. Section 4.4 discusses a methodology for determining a walker user's intent based on short-term goals (derived from a system dynamics model that maps force/moment input patterns to real-world actions), environmental modeling (to refine goals into those that make the most "sense"), an uncertainty model, and a set of heuristics. Section 4.5 then discusses how this intent can be manifested in assistive control when it appears that the user needs help completing their desired task. Section 4.6 contains an experimental evaluation of an intelligent walker system built using these techniques, and Section 4.7 discusses conclusions and future work.

4.2 Related Work

This section discusses existing mobility aids and divides them into classes based on the location of the user relative to the device. Some aids are "ride-able", that is, the user is carried by the device with their center of gravity riding vertically over the device's center of gravity. Others are not ride-able, with the user and device having horizontally displaced centers of gravity. We develop a taxonomy of devices and discuss how they are traditionally used. We then discuss work on intelligent versions of those devices. Finally, we examine related work in domains of shared control and mobile robotics. In particular, we examine robotic sensing and control strategies because these form the basis of our investigation into appropriate walker control systems.

4.2.1 Mobility Aids

Mobility aids for the elderly can be classified into two distinct categories: those that support the user's center of gravity above their own and those that do not. Wheelchairs and scooters fall into the first class, whereas canes and walkers fall into the second. Figure 4.1 shows a classification of devices that is relevant in the discussion of user intent and shared control.

Mobility aids differ based on their target user group. Ride-able devices, such as wheelchairs, are prescribed to users with insufficient lower body strength to remain standing for long periods. Wheelchairs can be either manually propelled or electrically powered. Electric wheelchairs are typically used by those with insufficient upper body strength (or motor coordination) to propel a manual wheelchair. Manual wheelchairs, in contrast, are prescribed more often than powered wheelchairs because they are less expensive and provide a certain amount of exercise. An interesting hybrid is the push-rim-activated power assist wheelchair (PAPAW) [16].

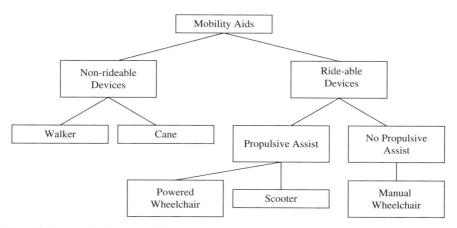

Fig. 4.1 A categorization of mobility aids

These wheelchairs use motors to augment the torque applied to the wheels by the user. Sensors in the wheel rims detect the torque being applied (how much, the differential between wheels) and control the motors to provide differential assist to the wheels based on the user's input and the situation. For example, a user without sufficient strength to propel a manual wheelchair up hill can use a PAPAW because it can augment the user's natural ability and provide sufficient force to move the chair up the incline. Scooters are another type of ride-able mobility aid that is widely used. Scooters are for persons with substantial upper body control, typically contain a swiveling seat and can be disassembled to fit into a vehicle such as a car [17]. However, the scooter's longer length typically means wider turning radii and thus more difficulty moving in home environments. In addition, scooters tend to be less customizable to the user's specific condition than powered wheelchairs. However, scooters are often substantially less expensive than powered wheelchairs and are a useful mobility aid, particularly outdoors.

A different class of mobility aids includes walkers, crutches, and canes. These aids are typically used more to assist in balance while ambulating and have been shown to reduce lower limb loads, increase biomechanical stability, and assist with initiation of the user's propulsion and braking during gait [18]. Canes have the advantage of being inexpensive and small (i.e., easy to transport, store, etc.) but provide asymmetric support when only one is used. Crutches, on the other hand, provide more symmetric support and are prescribed to prevent the loading one of the lower limbs.

Walkers are the second most commonly prescribed mobility aid after the cane [8]. However, walkers are prescribed in more disease processes and/or disabilities than any other mobility aid, with the four-legged "pick-up" walker being the most commonly prescribed. Despite their common use and prolonged existence, there are only a few studies in the literature that attempted to analyze the walker's use. One of these few attempts is the work of Fast et al. where strain gauges were mounted on all four legs of a walker to record forces transmitted through the walker's frame in axial, frontal, and sagittal orientations. The clinical testing of the instrumented walker on patients with ambulation dysfunction provided a better understanding of force distribution and revealed two distinct walker usage patterns. The first pattern was observed in patients using the walker as a means to reduce the amount of weight transmitted through the lower extremity. The second pattern was observed in patients with severe balance problems who used the walker to enhance their balance and stability [19]; finally, the walker could be used for a combination of weight support and balance enhancement. Walkers are available in a variety of configurations, including frame style walkers that contact the ground with four feet surrounding the user and must be lifted on each step. These walkers can be equipped with two or four skids or wheels instead of feet to allow the frame to be skidded or rolled on the floor for those with insufficient strength to repeatedly lift the frame. However, the wheels decrease the stability under weight-bearing conditions, and so, the use of wheels must be carefully considered. A different wheeled walker design, the "rollator," has three or four wheels with a built-in braking system allowing the walker to both roll and be held in place when necessary. These walkers also often have a seat that can be

Table 4.1 Information compiled from local survey of University of Virginia Health South facilities

Mobility aid — Disease process	Wheelchair	Walker/hemi-walker	Crutches/lofstrand crutches	Straight/quad cane
Cerebral palsy	X	X	X	
Parkinson's disease	X	X		X
Joint replacement		X		X
Lower extremity fractures		X	X	X
Peripheral neuropathies		X		X
Stroke/intracranial hemorrhage	X	X		X
Status post-neurosurgical procedures (aneurysm clipping, tumor resection)	X	X		X
Multiple trauma	X	X	X	X
Spinal cord injury, spine surgery	X	X		X
Multiple sclerosis	X	X		X

flipped down to allow the walker to be used as a chair when the user tires. Table 4.1 lists common conditions that require mobility aids and together with the potential types of mobility aids that could be prescribed for each of these conditions.

4.2.2 Intelligent Mobility Aids

While traditional mobility aids have definite advantages, several generations of intelligent mobility aids have expanded the utility and potential user population of these aids. Much of the early work on intelligent mobility aids utilized the wheelchair platform [2–7,20,21] (see [6] for a review of several projects). Typically, a commercially available powered wheelchair is modified to add environmental sensors and computer control. A number of control modes are available to assist the user with various situations, obstacle avoidance, wall following, door (opening) passage, and docking (intentionally approaching an object such as pulling up next to a table). Environmental sensors consist of sonar [21], cameras [2], and laser scanner [22] though many use a combination [3].

Commercial intelligent wheelchairs have also begun to appear. Although many have grown out of the above projects and are designed to assist in wheelchair navigation, the iBot [23] is an interesting exception. This wheelchair's main feature is its ability to achieve active balance on two wheels and therefore the ability to safely lift the user to the eye level of another (standing) person, carry users up stairs, and traverse uneven terrain that is usually considered too rough for other powered wheelchairs.

Intelligent walkers and canes have also been studied. Smart canes [24–27] have been developed as aids for the blind or visually impaired. These canes are actually wheeled devices which, unlike traditional canes, are not lifted off the floor on each step. Instead, they consist of a small wheeled base that rests on the floor and a long handle that extends up to the user's hand. The user interacts with the robot through the handle either directly through forces applied on the handle [26], through a small joystick at the end of the handle [24, 25], or through switches and a head-mounted gyroscope [27]. These canes create maps of the local environment (typically using sonar and/or cameras) and then use them to guide the user based on the user's desired destination input. However, all of these canes were designed as devices to guide the visually impaired. As such, they are not designed to handle the stability needs of the elderly. In fact, their somewhat large footprint can cause the user to stand farther away from their point-of-contact with the floor than they would with a traditional cane. This can significantly limit the robotic cane's weight-bearing ability. A related device is the Segway [28], a commercially available, two-wheeled mobility aid capable of carrying one person while standing. This device is not suitable for most elderly users with balance and stability issues because the Segway is controlled by the user leaning in the direction they wish to move. This intentional shifting of the user's center of gravity can be difficult/dangerous for users because it can destabilize them.

Intelligent walkers have recently begun to emerge as an alternative mobility aid to wheelchairs and scooters. Starting with the work of Lacey [29] on the PAM-AID (and later Guido [30]) projects, walkers have increasingly been studied [26, 31–33]. These walkers are modified rollator-style walkers with powered wheels and environmental sensors. They receive input from their user either through explicit control switches, dials, potentiometers or through force sensors connected to the walker's handles or steering column. Most of these walkers are designed for the frail, visually impaired and are meant to translate the user's "high-level" goals into navigation controls for the walker (which the user will then follow). An exception is the COOL-Aide [33–35], which is designed to operate in a more tightly coupled, shared control loop with its human user. Instead of active guidance, the COOL-Aide provides a passive, shared control system that delivers active steering assistance only as needed and no propulsion assistance—allowing the user to operate the walker as a normal walker at other times. One of the project's goals is to make the walker's assistance "invisible" in the sense that if assistance comes at the correct time, in judicious amounts, the user will be unaware that any assistance was provided. This is meant to provide a feeling of being in control instead of the feeling of being "lead."

4.3 COOL-Aide's Shared Control: Philosophy and Architecture

Shared control for intelligent mobility aids is unique due to the needs of its user community. In this section, we discuss the philosophy and system architecture of the COOL-Aide (CO-Operative Locomotion Aide) project, an intelligent walker for the elderly. COOL-Aide's philosophy of shared control is based on the following tenets:

1. The user is an integral part of the control system—The human operator of the walker is expected to be a continuous source of input. The user is not simply accepting or rejecting actions that the walker wishes to take but is always providing some direction to the walker/human system in addition to the propulsive force.

2. User intent is expressed in a natural way—The user provides input to the walker by using it in the same way that they would use a traditional ("non-intelligent") walker. This allows use of the device with no training and no additional cognitive load. The walker system's job is to assess the user's goals based on this input. While there is utility in explicit user input methods that allow direct expression of high-level goals, such as switches or voice input, the COOL-Aide project has focused on continuous navigational input and a more bottom-up synthesis of user intent. While such natural input is important in respecting a user's moment-to-moment navigation, providing the feeling of control and making the device easy to use, mobility aids may well benefit from a combination of both types of input methods.

3. The system should use passive control—Passive control means that the control system is not actively propelling the walker but only actively steering the walker when it deems necessary to act. The control system only activates in situations where the user needs assistance and de-activates after the situation has passed. This principle of providing "a little help when needed" is crucial in designing mobility aids for a large audience. In other words, we believe that there are a large number of people who can benefit from a small amount of assistance. Designs that focus on complex actuation or conceive of the mobility aid as "an autonomous robots that the user can lean on" have the potential to be discarded by the user populations especially if the users feel the aids are too restrictive (or controlling). Lack of use of prescribed mobility aids is already a major problem among the elderly [36].

4. The walker system's understanding of its user's intent can and will be incorrect at times. No system that determines its user's intent without explicit input of the user's goals will always make the correct assessment. Users can change their goals in the middle of a task or they can provide "noisy" input (e.g., dodging an obstacle on the way to their goal). A shared control system must be able to detect that its assessment of the user's intent has diverged from the user's actual intent and be able to take the appropriate action accordingly.

This philosophy has lead to the COOL-Aide architecture shown in Fig. 4.2.

The three boxes on the left represent the sensory input sub-systems. Each of these feeds into the key component for mapping natural human input into user intent, the system dynamics model. The output of this model is used, along with a map of the environment, to produce a list of probable user intents (goals). These intents, in turn, are used as input to the system's control logic that ultimately decides whether and how to operate the walker's steering motor. The control logic must also incorporate

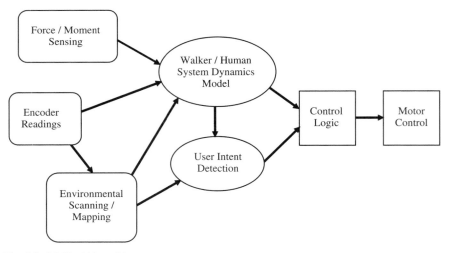

Fig. 4.2 COOL-Aide architecture

system dynamics (which describes how the walker would respond to propulsive and steering forces/moments) because some user intents may be inconsistent with maintaining user stability. The operation of each sub-system will be described in more detail in Section 4.4.

The COOL-Aide platform, shown in Fig. 4.3, is based on an Invacare three-wheeled walker frame. The force/moment sensing is performed by two six-axis force/moment sensors (ATI® US120-160/Mini45) mounted on the walker's handles

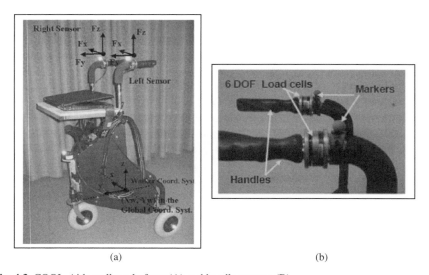

(a)   (b)

Fig. 4.3 COOL-Aide walker platform (A) and handle sensors (B) (as shown in part B of Fig. 4.3). The heading of the front steering wheel relative to the walker frame is measured using a 360° optical absolute position encoder (the A2 from US Digital®) mounted above the front wheel while the velocity of the back wheels is measured using two optical incremental encoders mounted on the axes of the rear wheels (the E5S model from US Digital®). The environmental sensing is performed with a 180° light-weight low-power infrared range-finding scanner (the PBS-03JN from Hokuyo Automation®). This scanner produces a radial depth map of a 3 m × 2 m area in front of the walker [37]. The walker can steer its front wheel relative to the frame through a stepper motor and controller (the PK296B2A-SG36 from Oriental Motors®). To eliminate the need to back-drive the stepper when the walker's control system is inactive, an electromagnetic clutch is used to connect the stepper to the front wheel (DetranPT® CS-22-B-24). The system is powered by a 24-V nickel metal hydride (Ni-MH) battery pack, and the walker's software runs on a 1.8 GHz Pentium® 4 laptop computer.

4.4 Assessing User Intent in COOL-Aide

The COOL-Aide system is designed to be used just as any other walker—the user simply pushes it where they want to go. Although this is perhaps the most natural interface, it requires the walker's control system to understand its user's intent based a stream of sensory data from various inputs over time. This section describes how the sensor data gathered by the walker is synthesized into a notion of the user's intent.

The COOL-Aide determines the user's intent through three main components: a dynamics model of the walker system that is used to predict the walker's path based on force/moment input, a model of the environment built from the IR scanner and encoder data, and an evidence-based uncertainty model that uses heuristic rules to combine information from the first two components into possible goals intended by the user. This model is implement on the basis of Dempster–Shafer theory.

4.4.1 A System Dynamics Model

The most important tool used in obtaining the user's intent is a physics-based mathematical model built to represent the walker's dynamics (i.e., how the walker moves in response to forces and moments). This two-dimensional dynamic model is a nonlinear, coupled set of differential equations built involving two rigid bodies: the walker frame and the front caster wheel, with the assumption that walker moves in planar space. The model converts three-dimensional force/moment input from the handles into the resulting direction of travel for the walker frame and the ground reaction force on each of the walker's wheels. The later output, principally influenced by the downward force the user places on the walker, is used in the computation of friction between the walker's wheels and the ground and hence to judge the likely speed of the walker. This friction computation also allows the model to account for sliding. This model was validated by experiments conducted in the Gait Lab of University of Virginia using data from a total of eight participants, three of whom were older adults (above 65). The detailed dynamic model of the walker is presented [34] along with its complete derivation method.

In addition to the walker's motion, the model outputs the stability margin of the walker frame using the principle of force-angle stability [38]. This stability measure accounts for the vertical load distribution on the walker and the effect of angular loads particularly moments about the axes of the walker's left and right sides. The value of the stability margin indicates the stability of the walker platform, which obviously impacts the stability of the walker user. The stability margin is used in evaluating the performance of the walker as discussed in Sections 4.5 and 4.6.

4.4.2 Environmental Sensing

The COOL-Aide builds a map of its local environment using the histogramic in-motion mapping (HIMM) technique [39]. The infrared scanner reads 121 data points at 1.8° intervals. The inner 100 points are used to form a 180° arc in front of the walker platform in the range of 200 mm–3 m. The size of the HIMM grid cells is chosen to be 100 mm because this approximates the minimum size object that can be detected by the scanner (based on the distance between scan intervals at 3 m). Each scan produces a radial depth map that adds evidence to a local map. The map is built up over time by adding each scan to the previous map. The rear wheel encoders' readings at the start of each scan are used to compute the translation and orientation of the map, relative to the previous scan before they are combined. Each scan reading in the radial depth map adds evidence for the existence of an object in the grid cell of the map that corresponds to azimuth of the reading and the measured distance. In addition, evidence is added for free space in every grid cell along the scan line between the walker and the detected object. Detected objects are grown using the standard growth rate operator (GRO) [39] to reflect the uncertainty in any particular scan in the depth map. In addition, a decay function is used to reduce occupancy evidence associated with any cell in the grid map (either for or against the presence of an object). This function's effect is to, over time, move every cell in the map that is not within range of the scanner toward the "unknown" state. Details about the parameters used in the mapping system are presented in reference [40].

4.4.3 Intent Heuristics and Uncertainty Model

Based on the output of the system dynamics model discussed in Section 4.4.1, a prediction of the walker's path over a 2-s time horizon is generated. Two seconds is chosen because this period was typically observed to give sufficient path predication to provide relatively smooth control actions (if necessary) while keeping the prediction error in an acceptable range [33]. The predicted path from the system dynamics model is then analyzed within the context of the environmental map discussed in Section 4.4.2. An uncertainty model based on Dempster–Shafer theory [41] was developed to weigh the likelihood of various possible user intents. This model assigns each "possible intent" a "possibility value" reflecting the system's belief that it is the user's actual intent. This possibility value (actually a tuple) is determined by analyzing the predicted path within the environment and the combining multiple of such analyses over time. The possibility computation involves some heuristic rules such as

- Passageways between objects in the environment are important positions for the walker to monitor. This is because small passageways can be difficult to navigate and so the control system is more likely to be activated in such a location than if the user were in an open area. All gaps between objects sufficiently large for the walker to safely go through, but less than 1.5 m wide, are considered as potential intended goals. Typically, a line between the closest points to the walker of the left and right obstacles that form the gap is drawn; the center of this line is used as the potentially intended goal location.

For each possible passageway, a 3-tuple is computed (possibility of passing through the passage, possibility of not passing through the passage, and possibility that the walker does not know the user's intent with respect to this passage). The first two possibility values are computed based on (i) how close the predicted path is to the possible goals (the closer the predicted path to the possible passageway, the more likely the user is attempting to go through it) and (ii) the distance to the possible passageway (the farther the goal is from the walker's current location, the more likely that the user is not trying to pass through that passageway); the third tuple element: value is 1 − (1st element + 2nd element).

Currently, correspondence between passageways identified in maps built from different scans is handled by simple nearest neighbor though a more robust system might be needed. The tuples computed for each possible goal are combined with evidence from previous local maps/path predictions using standard Dempster–Schafer rules [41]. A goal whose possibility tuple has a first element greater than 0.9 will be considered as the user's actual intent. Note that the system actively maintains the probabilities of multiple intents at all times, and so when one intent is determined to be invalid, the next most likely intent can be used by the control system instead.

4.5 COOL-Aide's Shared Control Based on User Intent

Broadly, the control system must make two decisions: (i) whether to actively control the walker's steering wheel or not and (ii) how to exactly control it. In general, providing active control as soon as possible (with respect to a particular user intent) allows the walker the greatest time horizon in which to operate and therefore allows for the smaller movements and hence results in smoother control. Although small movements of the wheel create less of a destabilizing effect, taking control actions too far away from the user's intended goal may contribute to a feeling that the user is not in control of the walker. In general, the user intent detection system's confidence in any particular goal is proportional to that goal's proximity to the walker, and so acting too early could result in the walker taking the wrong action (i.e., an action based on the wrong intent). Because of the affinity of the user intent detection system for physically close goals, the control system itself needs to perform little additional filtering on likely intents to decide whether to act when the intent detection system identifies a likely goal, the control system will begin to respond.

The control system receives three inputs: the user's goal from the intent detection system, a virtual moment from the obstacle avoidance system, and a signal from a module that analyses the instantaneous force/moment input to determine whether the user is resisting any current active control. The control system must then arbitrate between these signals to determine commands to send to the walker's motor. This arbitration proceeds as follows:

- Priority is given to responding to the user resisting control, then passage guidance and finally obstacle avoidance.
- If the user is not resisting control and a passageway is shown to be a goal by the user intent system, the control system begins active guidance control to guide the walker through the identified passageway.
- If the user is not resisting control and there is no passageway shown to be the user's intent, the control system will respond to the virtual moment provided by the obstacle avoidance system (see below) if needed.
- If the user is resisting control and the control system is performing active guidance, the control system will shift to obstacle avoidance control.
- If the user is resisting and the control system is performing obstacle avoidance, the control system will release active control (returning to passive mode and allowing the user to steer without any intervention from the system).

These rules have several interesting properties. The first is that the user will be allowed to possibly collide with an obstacle if they resist active attempts to avoid it by the walker. This is because the walker gives user control higher priority over its own active control. Through our research, it was found that users typically recognize what the walker is trying to do (avoid an obstacle) when the controller made the "correct" decision and follow the active control. When the controller makes the "wrong" decision, for example, avoiding an object that the user wishes to dock with, the user typically quickly resists the control decisions. The second property is that guidance through passageways has higher priority than obstacle avoidance. This is unusual in the mobile robotics community, where obstacle avoidance typically has higher priority than other goal-directed behaviors. However, COOL-Aide has a human user as an integral part of the control loop, and humans generally view objects in the environment as potential docking targets goals (a chair to sit in, a cabinet to open, a sink to use etc.) first and as obstacles to avoid second.

Once the control system decides on a control mode, it must select appropriate motor commands. Obstacle avoidance is performed in the following manner. Each object in the environment (within a certain radius) exerts a virtual repulsive moment on the walker proportional to the walker's proximity to that object [34]. The sum of these moments determines the resultant moment applied to the walker to turn it away from obstacles (so objects will "push" the walker away). To preserve the stability of the walker platform (and hence the user), the maximum virtual moment that can be applied is limited by the average stability index of the user (see the discussion of average stability in experiment 3 of Section 4.6.3). In other words, the obstacle avoidance system will turn the walker safely, where the turning radius is based on a stability measure calculated for each individual user. If passageway guidance is activated, the control system continuously calculates the wheel angle that will take the walker from its current position straight through the passageway. The wheel is turned to this angle and then held in place by activating all of the stepper motor's coils. The wheel angle is adjusted (and then held again) as need be as the actual movements of the walker are governed by both its wheel angle and the force/moment placed on it by the user. When the goal location is passed (typically determined using rear wheel IR sensors that detect, e.g., passing through the edges of doorways), the wheel is released and control is returned to the user.

Detecting that the user is resisting control occurs by performing two separate analyses on the force/moment input. First, the control system checks for large instantaneous changes in the moments exerted on the walker (>10Nm). Second, the control system checks for changes of more than 4 Nm in a sliding window of 10 samples. If either of these events occurs during active control, the user is considered to be resisting, and the walker's control is totally released to the user; this complies with the principle that the walker should help its user when it can but not impede them otherwise.

4.6 Preliminary Experimental Evaluation of COOL-Aide

To evaluate the walker's user intent detection and control system, a set of experiments were performed. Although preliminary, these experiments are unique in defining important quantitative criteria for evaluating intelligent mobility aids. Future work (involving more rigorous, long-term experiments with different/larger subject populations) will help clarify and refine issues discovered during this evaluation. The experiments measure the walker's ability to detect user intent, avoid obstacles, provide pro-active guidance, and detect/resolve conflict between the user's intent and the walker's assessment of the user's intent. This section describes the experimental setup, subject population, and experimental outcomes.

4.6.1 Experimental Setup

All experiments were performed in the University of Virginia's Motor Performance Lab at the Kluge Children's Rehabilitation Center (KCRC). The actual movements of walker were recorded by a VICON® 612 motion capture system using six 120-Hz video cameras. Eight reflective markers were placed on the walker and

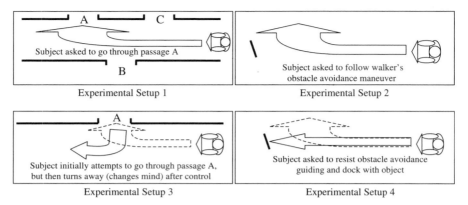

Fig. 4.4 Experimental setups for walker evaluation

6 more were placed on objects in the environment. The positions of these sensors in a global coordinate frame were recorded by the motion capture system. The data from the walker's sensors, including force/moment data, encoder readings, and environmental maps were also recorded. Experimental results are determined by post-processing the data to determine how well the "ground truth" movement of the walker, as measured by the motion capture system, corresponded to the walker system's desired outcome.

A series of four experiments were performed with each experiment being carried out by each subject three times. The environmental layouts for the experiments are shown in Fig. 4.4. In each experiment, the subject was asked to push the walker and perform various maneuvers. To simulate the walking speed of an elderly user with mobility issues, subjects were asked to walk at approximately 0.5 m/s (shown through demonstration). This corresponds to a speed slightly slower than the walking speed of normal adults (0.7 m/s [13]).

Two experiments were performed using experimental setup 1. Experiment 1 was designed to test the walker's ability to determine user's intent, and so no active control was provided. A set of obstacles was set up with three openings, labeled A, B, and C in Fig. 4.4—experimental setup 1. The subject was asked to push the walker through the opening labeled A, and the walker's determination of the user's intent over time was recorded. Specifically, the number of times the user intent detection loop correctly or incorrectly detected the "go through A" intent and the time it took the system to determine the intent were measured. Experiment 2 was designed to evaluate the walker's proactive guidance. In this experiment, the user was asked to push the walker through passage A, as before, while the walker provided assistive steering as needed this time. The offset between the center of the passage and the point at which the walker's midline actually crossed the passage opening were measured.

Experiment 3 involved the walker's stability-based obstacle avoidance. Using the environment shown in experimental setup 2, the user was asked to push the walker at an obstacle and then follow when the walker tried to maneuver away from it.

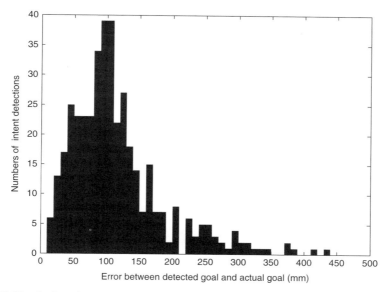

Fig. 4.5 Distribution of errors between detected user intent and actual user intent

Although the walker may detect the obstacle at a large distance (2–3 m away), it will not perform any maneuver until it determines from the user's intent is that the user will impact the obstacle. At this point, it will activate control. However, the obstacle avoidance algorithm considers the stability of the walker platform (which is used as an indicator of the stability of the human) and so will turn safely. The mean and standard deviation of the distance between the walker and the obstacle, as well as the number of obstacle impacts were measured.

A third set of experiments was performed to evaluate the walker's ability to detect and resolve conflicts between the user's actual intent and the walker's assessment of this intent. Experiment 4 was performed using experimental setup 3, in which the user was asked to initially head for passage A and then turn away after proactive control activates. This was to simulate a situation where the walker incorrectly determined the user's intent or the user simply changed their mind. Experiment 5, performed using experimental setup 4, involved the user moving toward an obstacle as in experiment 3; however, when the walker controller attempted to avoid the obstacle, the user was instructed to resist and instead try and dock with the object. For both experiments 4 and 5, the time between the instance the user began to show a different intent (determined in post-processing of the handle force time series) and the instance at which the walker detected that the user's current input does not match the walker's intent assessment was measured.

The experiments were conducted under Institutional Review Board (IRB) approval.

4.6.2 Characteristics of Subjects

Twelve subjects (10 males and 2 females) evaluated the walker. Eight of the subjects were healthy adults while four subjects had disorders that affected their mobility. Three subjects had cerebral palsy and one had familial torsion dystonia (DYS). The mean age of subjects was mean ± SD; the subjects' age and gender appear in Table 4.2. The healthy subjects performed all of the experiments described in Section 4.6.1, whereas the four subjects with mobility disorders performed only user intent detection experiment 1 due to concerns about their stamina during a longer suite of tests.

In Table 4.2, H denotes a healthy subject, CP denotes a subject with cerebral palsy, and DYS denotes a subject with familial torsion dystonia. The final four subjects were selected because it is believed that the walker's technology while designed for the elderly, could also be of use to children (adolescents) with pathological mobility issues. The walker platform has not been evaluated yet on elderly subjects with mobility issues and will be evaluated in the near future.

4.6.3 Preliminary Experimental Results

The primary aim of the COOL-Aide project was to determine user intent based on natural input. To this end, Experiment 1 is perhaps the most important. Between experiments 1 and 2, 40 trials were conducted using the healthy subjects (24 "pure" user intent-detection trials and 16 trials including active guidance). Each of these trials utilized the walker's ability to detect user intent, and the results are summarized in Fig. 4.5.

From Fig. 4.5, we can see that the most common error is on the order of 100 mm (the two largest bins in the histogram are for 100 and 110 mm). In fact, 242 of 410 detections (59%) had errors of 110 mm or less. The maximum error approaches 500 mm. However, this seemingly large error may be mitigated by several factors. First, the detected goal location is not directly used for control. In other words, the walker does not simply head for the detected goal location but instead scans in the environment for other information that might allow refinement of that goal. In this case, the "actual" goal location is defined as the center point between the two edges of passage A. If the detected goal is somewhere within passage A, that detection will contribute strong evidence to trigger the control to guide the user through passage A. During these experiments, all errors were small enough to activate passage guidance control (see the discussion below on the success of that control).

Table 4.2 Characterization of subjects

Subject #	1	2	3	4	5	6	7	8	9	10	11	12
Age	36	60	38	52	41	33	65	52	21	14	14	15
Gender	M	M	M	M	M	F	M	M	M	M	F	M
Physical condition	H	H	H	H	H	H	H	H	CP	CP	CP	DYS

Table 4.3 User intent-detection timing

Time to detect user's intent	Healthy subjects (40 trials)	CP and DYS subjects (10 trials)
Mean (s)	0.4403	0.9059
Standard deviation (s)	0.5055	1.0024

The walker uses an evidence-based system for computing user's intent. Therefore, intents are not recognized instantaneously but instead need time for enough evidence to be accumulated. The time to accumulate this evidence was measured and is summarized in Table 4.3. Note that this is the time from the first instantaneous intent detection (which the control system would not respond to) until enough evidence for that intent had been gathered such that the control system would respond (if required).

For experiment 2, the user's intent over time was assessed by the walker's control system and the walker's estimates of the desired goal locations were plotted. Figure 4.6 shows an example trial from an overhead perspective. The large triangles represent positions of the walker frame over time as captured by the motion capture system. Asterisks ("*") indicate the position of the walker when the control system had enough information to predict the user's intent. The crosses ("+") indicate predicted goals, and the lines connect intent detection (star) to the corresponding predicted goal (cross). Note that, for clarity, only detected intents that required the walker to perform a guidance action are shown. In other words, at the beginning

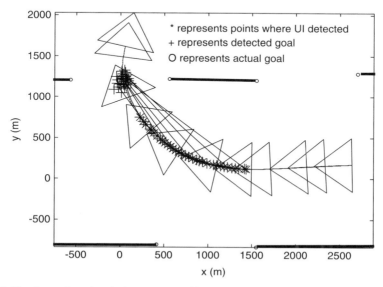

Fig. 4.6 User intent detection during passage guidance

of the trial, the detected user intent is to proceed straight down the hallway. However, as the hall passageway is wide (and therefore not difficult to navigate), the control system initially remained passive and therefore this intent is not reflected in Fig. 4.6. Also, for clarity, the position of the walker (triangle) is only plotted every 10 samples. The actual intended goal of the user is given to the subjects by the experimenter ("go through passage A"). However, the exact point in space that the user heads for was not precisely defined. We define a correct intent detection as the walker's estimate of the goal location being within 0.2 m of the point in the middle of the passage, along a line parallel to the wall. This value was chosen because it corresponds to the expected error in the size of objects in the environmental map based on the map's cell size (0.1 m) and the GRO operator used (which adds an additional 0.1 m).

The effectiveness of the active guidance was measured by comparing the location of the walker's center line when it passed through the passage with the actual centerline of the opening (termed the offset distance). For the 16 trials with active guidance, the results are shown in the histogram of Fig. 4.7.

While none of the 16 trials had an *offset* too great to facilitate passage of the 1.1 m passage used in experiment 2 (though other factors limited success—see below), standard interior doors are less than 1 m wide. This means that, given the difference between the width of the walker and a standard 0.9144 m (36") interior door, an offset of more than 100 mm will not allow passage. A more robust control algorithm will likely be necessary to deal with these smaller openings. A more serious issue is that two of the 16 trials did not clear the passage because the walker approached the passage from too acute an angle. In other words, while the walker's center and the door passage's center were physically close, the angle of approach made it difficult to easily turn the walker through the door without impacting

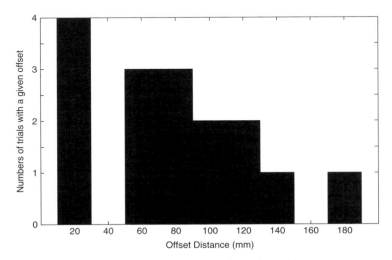

Fig. 4.7 Offset between walker and passage centers during active guidance

the door frames. In general, approaching a passageway from an acute angle is a difficult control problem. The user should first be guided away from the passage to allow for an entry angle close to 90°, but this may prove confusing and may require higher turning rates that may be considered unsafe. Another alternative is to turn sharply when the walker is in the correct position, instead of making the gentler turn that a less shallow angle affords. However, sharp turns have a greater destabilizing effect. More sophisticated control strategies may be needed to improve the performance. As the COOL-Aide is controlled by both the user and the computer and is designed to prioritize user stability, it may not be able to successfully navigate all scenarios. In other words, COOL-Aide is not an autonomous robot that should be expected to operate without human intervention. Instead it relies on its user to be an integral part of the control of the walker/human system. If the walker cannot successfully navigate a passage (although it maintains user stability), control should be transferred back to the user—allowing them to perhaps back up and readjust their position and angle of entry.

Experiment 3 attempted to understand how active control affects user stability. To this end, we define a stability index for the walker platform based on tipping moments [42] about the two axes for the left and right sides of the walker (see Figure 4.3). This index is a unit-less quantity in which higher numbers indicate more stability. It should be noted that the stability of the walker platform is not a perfect indicator of the stability of the human [38]. In general, if the walker is unstable, the human user is very likely to also be unstable. But, the human may be unstable while the walker platform remains stable, for example, when falling over backwards. However, walker stability can be measured online based on force/moment input from the handle sensors, whereas a general measure of human stability requires sensing of all the human's joint angles.

The "normal" stability of each user was calculated by having them lean their weight on the walker and push the walker forward several meters. This was repeated three times and an average value of the individuals' stability index was computed. This value was then used as a threshold during stability-based obstacle avoidance. If the stability of the walker dropped below the individualized threshold, the walker ceased any active control it was taking (under the assumption that the walker was, e.g., turning too hard). Table 4.4 shows the mean and standard deviation for the minimum distance between the walker and obstacles during the 42 trials in the cases of both the obstacle avoidance control algorithm that considered stability index as a constraint during obstacle avoidance and the algorithm that did not incorporate the stability index as a constraint.

Two issues emerge from Table 4.4. The first is that the mean distance by which the walker cleared obstacles is lower when stability was taken into account. This is because the walker generally makes smoother turns (at lower turning rates) and therefore follows a longer arc to avoid objects when the stability index was incorporated as a constraint into the obstacle avoidance control algorithm. The second issue is the number of times that the walker actually impacted the obstacle, that is, failed to avoid it. The walker's obstacle avoidance system was designed bearing in mind that it is more important to maintain stability than to avoid obstacles

Table 4.4 Performance of obstacle avoidance with and without user stability preservation

	Minimum distance between walker and obstacle during successful obstacle avoidance		Percentage of trials with obstacle contact
	Mean (mm)	Standard deviation (mm)	
"Standard" obstacle avoidance	230.86	108.87	0 (0/26)
Stability preserving obstacle avoidance	96.02	73.58	43.75 (7/16)

(given the generally low speed of impact). However, it was found that user's typical initial response to active control by the walker was to loosen their grip on the walker's handles. This caused the stability index to drop below the individualized threshold and therefore to de-activate the control. Then the user would tend to take over again and continue pushing toward the obstacle, as they had been instructed. While subsequent attempts by the walker to avoid the obstacle did not elicit the same reaction (and therefore drop in stability), the walker had, in many cases, come too close to the object too, and with the constraint on the turning rate, it was unable to turn sharply enough to avoid it. This user's behavior indicated that the new control mode introduced nuances that could be overcome with training the users, and that while the human/walker dynamics model works well when the walker is passive, the model may require refinement to handle the human/machine feedback loop when the walker's control is active.

Experiments 4 and 5 were designed to evaluate the walker's ability to detect that it has identified the wrong user intent. The walker system constantly tracks multiple possible user intents, by assigning each a probability and updating the probabilities regularly based on new information available to the system. The most likely intent is the one that has a high enough probability to potentially activate the control system. In experiment 4, the user was asked to switch intents during the trial by first heading to passage A and then veering away. In experiment 5, the walker tries to avoid the object that the user wishes to dock with, thus creating a conflict of intent between the control system and the user. The time from when the walker first activates control appropriate to the identified intent until the walker recognizes the correct intent is measured in seconds and summarized in Table 4.5.

Table 4.5 Time to detect that user's intent does not match intent on which control is based

	Time to detect new intent during passage guidance (experiment 4)	Time to detect new intent during obstacle avoidance (experiment 5)	Time to detect intent "conflict" based on instantaneous moment	Time to detect intent "conflict" based on sliding window
Mean (s)	1.773	1.699	1.555	1.768
Standard deviation (s)	1.047	0.544	0.512	1.014

The walker uses two different methods to analyze user force/moment input to determine when a user's intent differs from the intent that is currently driving the control system. Both methods are used simultaneously. The first method looks for large (10 Nm), instantaneous changes in the moment exerted on the handles by the user. This corresponds to the increased torque necessary to steer the walker in a direction other than the one the control is pursuing. The second method looks for gradual resistance to a control steering action by examining a sliding window of 10 samples from the force/moment sensors. An average moment of 4 Nm within this window indicates that the user is resisting the walker's control over time (though less strongly than in the "instantaneous" case). The first two columns of Table 4.5 show the time taken to detect a change in user intent during different control maneuvers. The second two columns show the time taken to detect an intent change using the two detection methods (i.e., the time necessary to trigger one criterion or the other). There are two potential issues with large conflict detection times. First is that the walker could cause the user to travel along the wrong path for some distance, with longer detection times causing divergence form the user's intended goal and thus making the attainment of the goal more difficult. The second issue is the user's feeling/perception of the system's control actions based on incorrect intent. If the detection time is too long, users may feel that they are laboring to get the device to go where they want; thus, they may be frustrated and may release their grip on the device not understanding the walker's seemingly incorrect behavior. While it remains an open question how problematic "following the wrong path" may be, comments from users who participated in these trials indicate that the "feeling of control" issue was being raised by these detection times. Further research into detection methods and faster sensing mechanisms (which form the lower bound on detection time) are needed.

4.7 Conclusions

Intelligent mobility aids have the potential to impact a larger population than ever before. By increasing the ease and safety of daily mobility tasks, the users' ability to perform ADLs and IADLs can be significantly improved. In addition, mobility aids may increase the time during which a user can live independently, thereby reducing the overall cost of long-term care. The ability of users to gain access to this technology is increasing as well, as many intelligent mobility aids are beginning to leave research labs and enter the commercial market. Projects, such as COOL-Aide, have shown the merit of natural interfaces to intelligent mobility aids. Such interfaces are easy to use and learn. In our tests, users did not require training or instruction on the use of COOL-Aide nor did they have difficulty using it (including CP patients with significant mobility issues).

However, more development work is needed particularly in the refinement of the control system. One promising avenue is to factor in the user's gait cycle which can be detected through the force/moment sensors [31]. Oscillating patterns in the input streams from the left and right force sensors on the walker's handles can allow the detection of heel strikes for the left and right feet. It is hoped that this information could make active control more transparent to the user by, for example, only adjusting the wheel in a particular direction when the left foot is on the ground (and similarly for the right foot). In addition, increased user stability might be achieved by only having control active during the user's double support phase (when both feet are on the ground). Another interesting possibility is to use the walker outside the lab gait monitor, recording/analyzing gait parameters during the user's regular use throughout the day. Such longitudinal gait monitoring capability could shed light on not only how user's gait changes over time, both as a consequence of the natural aging process or the onset of a disease condition, but also the effect and efficacy of interventions including the mobility aid itself.

The field of intelligent mobility aids, involving both design and evaluation, is an exciting, cross-disciplinary field. Intelligent wheelchairs have had many years of design, evaluation and refinement. Intelligent walkers, however, are just beginning large-scale testing. The COOL-Aide's results, while preliminary, show promise, and work is ongoing both on walkers designed for elderly adults and walker designed for children with cerebral palsy. Although the underlying gait issues may differ between these populations, the underlying science of shared control based on user intent detection is applicable to different populations.

Acknowledgments This material is based upon work supported by the National Science Foundation under grant no. 0139283. Any opinions, findings, and conclusions or recommendations expressed in this material are those of the authors and do not necessarily reflect the views of the National Science Foundation.

References

1. Njegovan, V., et al. 2001. The hierarchy of functional loss associated with cognitive decline in older persons. *Journal of Gerontology*, 56A (10), M638–M643.
2. Gomi, T., Ide, K. 1996. The development of an intelligent wheelchair. *Proceedings of the IEEE Intelligent Vehicle Symposium*, pp. 70–75.
3. Gribble, W., et al. 1998. Integrating vision and spatial reasoning for assistive navigation. In V. Mittal, H. Yanco, J. Aronis and R. Simpson (eds), *Assistive Technology and Artificial Intelligence, Lecture Notes in Computer Science*, Springer Verlag, New York, pp. 179–193.
4. KISS Institute for Practical Robotics. *The TinMan Supplemental Wheelchair Controller.* http://www.kipr.org/robots/tm.html. Accessed August 2006.
5. Mori, H., Kotani, S., Kiyohiro, N. 1998. HITOMI: design and development of a robotic travel aid. In Mittal et al. (eds.) *Lecture Notes in Artificial Intelligence: Assistive Technology and Artificial Intelligence*, Springer-Verlag, New York, pp. 221–234.
6. Simpson, R., et al. 2004. The smart wheelchair component system. *Journal of Rehabilitation Research and Development*, 41 (3B), 429–442.
7. Yanco, H. 1998. Wheelesley, a robotic wheelchair system: indoor navigation and user interface. In V.O. Mittal, H.A. Yanco, J. Aronis, and R. Simspon (eds), *Lecture Notes in Artificial Intelligence: Assistive Technology and Artificial Intelligence*, Springer-Verlag, New York, pp. 256–268.

8. National Center for Health Statistics. 1997. *Trends and Differential Use of Assistive Technology Devices: United States*. Vital and Health Statistics – Centers for Disease Control and Prevention, no. 292, November 13. http://www.cdc.gov/nchs/data/ad/ad292.pdf. Accessed September 19, 2007.

9. National Center for Health Statistics. 1997. *Frequencies of Activity Limitations among Persons 18 Years of Age or Older in the US*. http://www.cdc.gov/nchs/fastats/pdf/sr10_205t18.pdf. Accessed November 2006.

10. Administration on Aging. 2005. *A Profile of Older Americans 2005*. http://www.aoa.gov/PROF/Statistics/profile/2005/2005profile.pdf. Accessed November 2006.

11. Ciole R., Trusko, B. 1999. HealthCare 2020: challenges for the millennium. *Health Management Technology*, 20 (7):34–38.

12. US Census Bureau. 2002. *Global Population at a Glance: 2002 and Beyond*. http://www.census.gov/ipc/prod/wp02/wp02-1.pdf. Accessed August 2006.

13. Kramarow, E., et al. 1999. *Health and Aging Chartbook, Health United States, National Center for Health Statistics*. http://www.cdc.gov/nchs/data/hus/hus99.pdf. Accessed August 2006.

14. Yu, W., Ezzati-Rice, T. 2005. *Concentration of Health Care Expenditures in the U.S. Civilian Noninstitutionalized Population*. Statistical Brief #81. Agency for Healthcare Research and Quality. http://www.meps.ahrq.gov/papers/st81/stat81.pdf.

15. National Center for Injury Prevention. Hip Fractures among Older Adults. Centers for Disease Control. http://www.cdc.gov/ncipc/factsheets/fallcost.htm. Accessed September 19, 2007.

16. Cooper, R.A., et al. 2004. *Push For Power*. Rehab Management. http://www.rehabpub.com/features/32004/5.asp. Accessed August 2006.

17. Cooper, R.A., Cooper, R. 2003. *Trends and Issues in Wheeled Mobility Technologies*. Wheeled Mobility Workshop, October 9–11, Buffalo, NY.

18. Bateni, H., Maki, B. 2005. Assistive Devices for Balance and Mobility: Benefits, Demands, and Adverse Consequences. *Archives of Physical Medicine and Rehabilitation*, 86 (1):134–145.

19. Fast A., et al. 1995. The Instrumented Walker: Usage Patterns and Forces. *Archives of Physical Medicine and Rehabilitation*, 76950:484–491.

20. Nisbet, P., Craig, I. 1994. Mobility and mobility training for severely disabled children: results of the "Smart" Wheelchair project, *Proceedings of RESNA '94*, pp. 17–22.

21. Simpson, R., Levine, S. 1999. Automatic adaptation in the NavChair assistive WheelChair navigation system. *IEEE Transaction on Rehabilitation Engineering*, 7 (4):452–463.

22. Rofer, T. 2001. Building Consistent Laser Scan Maps. *4th European Workshop on Advanced Mobile Robots (EUROBOT-2001)*, 86:83–90.

23. iBot Mobility System. 2006. *Independence Technology*. http://www.independencenow.com/ibot/intro.html?from=ggl. Accessed August 2006.

24. Aigner, P., McCarragher, B. 1999. Shared control framework applied to a robotic aid for the blind. *IEEE Control Systems Magazine*, 19 (2):40–46.

25. Borenstein, J., Ulrich, I. 1997. *The Guidecane – A Computerized Travel Aid for the Active Guidance of Blind Pedestrians*. IEEE International Conference on Robotics and Automation Albuquerque, New Mexico, pp. 1283–1288.

26. Dubowsky, S., et al. 2000. PAMM – A Robotic Aid to the Elderly for Mobility Assistance and Monitoring: A "Helping-Hand" for the Elderly. *Proceedings of the IEEE International Conference on Robotics and Automation (ICRA 00)*, San Francisco, CA, 570–576.

27. Shim, I., Yoon, J., Yoh, M. 2004. A Human Robot Interactive System "RoJi". *International Journal of Control, Automation, and Systems*, 2 (3):398–405.

28. Segway Inc. 2006. http://www.segway.com. Accessed November 2006.

29. Lacey, G., Dawson-Howe, K. 1999. The application of robotics to a mobility aid for the elderly blind. *Robotics and Autonomous Systems*, 23:245–252.

30. GUIDO Smart Walker. 2006. Haptica Corporation. http://www.haptica.com/id2.htm. Accessed August 2006.

31. Alwan, M., et al. 2006. Basic Walker-assisted gait characteristics derived from forces and moments exerted on the Walker's handles: results on normal subjects. *Journal of Medical Engineering & Physics*, 29 (3):380–389.
32. Morris, A., et al. A Robotic Walker that Provides Guidance. *Proceedings of the 2003 IEEE Conference on Robotics and Automation (ICRA '03)*.
33. Wasson, G., et al. 2004. A Physics-Based Model for Predicting User Intent in Shared-Control Pedestrian Mobility Aids, *IEEE/RSJ International Conference on Intelligent Robots and Systems (IROS 04)*, pp. 1914–1919.
34. Huang, C. 2006. *User's Intent Detection and Shared Control: Application to an Intelligent Walker*. PhD Thesis, Department of Mechanical and Aerospace Engineering, University of Virginia.
35. Wasson, G., et al. 2003. User Intent in a Shared Control Framework for Pedestrian Mobility Aids. *IEEE/RSJ International Conference on Intelligent Robots and Systems (IROS 03)*, pp. 2962–2967.
36. Scherer, M., Galvin, J. 1994. Matching people with technology. *Rehabilitation Management*, 7 (2):128–130.
37. Alwan, M., et al. 2005. Characterization of Infrared Range-Finder PBS-03JN for 2-D Mapping, *International Conference on Robotics and Automation 205 (ICRA '05)*, pp. 3936–3941.
38. Alwan, M., et al. 2005. Stability Margin Monitoring in Steering-Controlled Intelligent Walkers for the Elderly, *AAAI Fall Symposium 2005: Caring Machines*.
39. Borenstein, J., Koren, Y. 1991. Histogramic in-motion mapping for mobile robot obstacle avoidance. *IEEE Transaction on Robotics & Automation*, 7 (4):535–539.
40. Huang, C., et al. 2005. Shared Navigational Control and User Intent Detection in an Intelligent Walker, *AAAI Fall Symposium 2005: Caring Machines*.
41. Shafer, G. 1976. *A Mathematical Theory of Evidence*. Princeton University Press, Princeton, NJ.
42. Papadopoulos, E., Rey, D. 2000. The force-angle measure of tipover stability margin for mobile manipulators. *Journal of Vehicle System Dynamics*, 33:29–48.

Chapter 5
Sleep and Sleep Assessment Technologies

Steven M. Koenig, David Mack, and Majd Alwan

5.1 Importance of Sleep Disorders and the Effects of Aging on Sleep

On average, we sleep about one-third of our lives. Sleep is something we do every-day; yet, it appears from the 2005 Sleep in America Poll conducted by the National Sleep Foundation (NSF) that while about 75% of Americans indicated that they have at least one symptom of a sleep disorder, the same survey indicates that 76% of Americans do not think they have a sleep problem and only 45% would report it to their doctor if they felt they had issues [1]. Although the people who voluntarily lose sleep can resolve their problem without treatment, 10–13% of Americans (30–40 million) are suffering from clinical sleep disorders that cause them to have disrupted sleep and, hence, affect their health [2]. Untreated sleep disorders lead to losses in productivity totaling around $46 billion annually in the USA, health problems including a higher risk for stroke, or even fatality, with an estimated 38,000 deaths annually attributed to complications from sleep apnea [3]. The condition of sleep apnea, or more broadly sleep-disordered breathing (SDB), is quite prevalent in the US population with at least 12 million Americans suffering from it [4] (Figure 5.1).

In 2003, the National Institutes of Health (NIH) released its latest Sleep Disorders Research Plan that outlines research to date in specific areas, but also lays out needs for additional work to be done to advance our understanding of sleep in those areas. As mentioned earlier, SDB, the most prevalent of which is obstructive sleep apnea (OSA), affects millions of Americans, and many of them do not undergo treatment because the condition remains formally undiagnosed [2]. OSA is quantified by counting events termed apneas (stoppages of breathing during sleep for at least 10 s) and hypopneas (an abnormal respiratory event with a decrease in respiratory effort

Steven M. Koenig

Professor of Internal Medicine, University of Virginia Health System, The Department of Internal Medicine, Division of Pulmonary & Critical Care, Box 800546, Charlottesville, VA 22908-0546

e-mail: smk4q@virginia.edu

From: *Aging Medicine, Eldercare Technology for Clinical Practitioners,*
Edited by: M. Alwan and R. Felder © Humana Press, Totowa, NJ

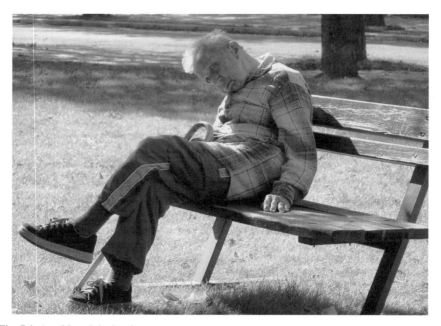

Fig. 5.1 An older adult sleeping

or airflow of at least 30% that lasts for at least 10 s) that may occur only a few times an hour in normal subjects or beyond 15 times per hour [5]. The standard therapy to treat SDB uses continuous positive airway pressure (CPAP) devices that are generally composed of a mask and an air pressure system that forces the airways to stay open during sleep. These tend to be cumbersome and expensive; yet, it can be the only way a subject with severe sleep apnea might be able to consistently sleep well [2].

Researchers are beginning to find clues as to the pathogenesis and possible genetic links to the condition of OSA along with other neurological modalities that cause airways to collapse during an apnea. More research needs to be conducted in higher numbers to continue to evaluate these findings and understand more about what causes OSA and how best to treat it. The NIH suggests that current methods for measuring breathing abnormalities are cumbersome, expensive, lack predictive power, and are useless for screening large populations. To accomplish this faster, in a wider population and more natural setting, the NIH states that researchers should "develop novel non-invasive screening/diagnostic methodologies that are less expensive and more widely applicable than standard full polysomnography" [2]. To further challenge sleep studies, there is no comprehensive database that defines normal sleep–wake patterns based on age or gender. As a result, the NIH identifies a need for new methods that can non-invasively monitor sleep and respiration to quantify breathing problems and their consequences [4].

In addition to the problems of sleep disorders such as OSA, sleep patterns and habits tend to change as people age. According to the NSF's 2003 Sleep in America Poll, which focused on the sleep of older adults, nearly half (48%) frequently have at least one symptom of insomnia. The main cause of the insomnia is related to waking up in the middle of the night and not being able to return to sleep. Part of this results from the nearly two-thirds of older adults (65%) who report having to get up to go to the bathroom at least a few nights a week [6]. This fragmentation of sleep leads to decreases in sleep quality and increases in daytime sleepiness. Some of the rise in the prevalence of these conditions can be attributed to independent factors associated with aging including bereavement of a loved one and mental health deterioration among others, but it is still clearly an important area of interest [2].

Sleep is needed to maintain physical, mental, and emotional health, [7] and the changes that occur in seniors over time with regard to their sleep can affect how well rested they are each day, on each of these levels. The NIH realizes the need for better understanding older adults' sleep problems and any role they may play in the cognitive decline, which could be crucial to unlocking secrets of dementia and Alzheimer's. Furthermore, the NIH sees the need to establish what is considered normal changes of sleep with age so that treatments can be properly targeted to people who need them the most [4]. Longitudinal studies, especially those centered on circadian patterns, are necessary to accomplish these goals, and new non-invasive technology acceptable for use in the home environment should be implemented to allow large-scale, long-term studies to be conducted in a natural setting. This objective data could give us a clear look at the sleep patterns and habits of older adults that could provide answers to some of these questions about cognitive decline and changes in sleep behavior.

The clinical gold standard of polysomnography (PSG), although highly detailed and thorough in its analysis of sleep, is not designed to effectively conduct studies on large scales. Additionally, it is not suited to operate over multiple nights in a person's natural environment, so new equipment needs to be developed to fulfill the need, as the NIH recognizes in their research plan. However, such new equipment and techniques must be validated against the existing clinical gold standard before it can be effectively used as a research or a clinical assessment tool.

The future of sleep research for now seems to be squarely focused on taking advantage of advances on technology so we might be able to learn more about something we do everyday. The NIH states this clearly in their research plan [2]:

> New approaches are needed for the measurement, assessment, and quantification of physiologic/biologic variables during sleep. Such methods should be easily accomplished to permit broad applicability, quantitative, and predictive of the consequences of the sleep disorder under assessment. The focus should be on novel, noninvasive approaches that do not require labor-intensive, expensive scoring, perhaps including microtechnology.

Time will tell what we will learn about sleep and its effects on our lives. For now, we must challenge ourselves to accept new ways of thinking about sleep research, yet compare those new ways to the gold standards that exist today.

5.2 The Sleep Health Heart Study

The Sleep Health Heart Study (SHHS) is a multicenter study of the cardiovascular consequences of sleep–SDB [8, 9]. It represents the largest cohort study to date of not only SDB but normal sleep as well. Studies analyzing the data thus far have contributed substantially to the field of sleep medicine in general and our understanding of SDB in particular.

Subjects for the SHHS were recruited from participants in ongoing population-based cohort studies of cardiovascular or respiratory disease in the USA. Exclusion criteria included age less than 40 years, treatment of sleep apnea with CPAP or an oral appliance, home oxygen therapy, and having a tracheotomy. Selection and recruitment procedures varied by study site. Because the sampling frame for the study already constituted a somewhat selected group, no effort was made to obtain a random sample. To optimize statistical power by increasing the prevalence of SDB in younger participants, for subjects younger than 65 years, those who reported snoring at least three nights per week (habitual snoring) were intentionally over sampled.

Among 11,053 participants in the parent cohorts who were potentially eligible, 6841 (62%) were enrolled for the SHHS baseline sleep study between November 1995 and January 1998. Before the baseline home visit and sleep study, participants completed a self-administered sleep habits questionnaire. The home visit included a brief health interview, blood pressure and anthropometric measurements, and a single night, unattended PSG using a portable monitor (Compumedics® P-2 System; Abbotsford, Australia). Of the 6841 home PSG studies attempted, 401 (5.9%) had less than 4 h of recorded data of sufficient quality to allow sleep staging and respiratory event detection. The remaining 6440 PSG studies were reviewed and scored at a central reading center (Case Western University, Cleveland, OH, USA). A detailed protocol for scoring of sleep stages, arousals, and respiratory events has been described [9, 10].

Data from the SHHS have revealed the following associations between SDB and cardiovascular and metabolic diseases. Nieto et al. demonstrated an association between two markers of the severity of SDB, the apnea–hypopnea index (AHI) and the percentage of sleep time <90% arterial oxygen saturation (SaO_2), and the prevalence of hypertension (see below for definitions) [11]. Shahar and colleagues [12] reported that even AHI values in the normal to mildly elevated range are associated with an increased risk of coronary heart disease, heart failure, and stroke. Mehra et al. [13] established that SDB is associated with an increased risk of arrhythmias including atrial fibrillation, non-sustained ventricular tachycardia, and complex ventricular ectopy. Finally, Punjabi and coworkers [14] noted that the average level of oxygen saturation-predicted insulin resistance in non-diabetic participants. Of note, and somewhat surprisingly, the study by Punjabi et al., as well as others in the medical literature, suggests that the cardiovascular consequences associated with SDB may be weaker in the elderly as compared with middle-aged adults. An intriguing possibility is that changes of the autonomic nervous system with aging may actually be protective in mitigating adverse cardiovascular responses to SDB-associated physiologic perturbations.

The SHHS has also contributed to our understanding of the non-cardiovascular, non-metabolic consequences of SDB such as excessive daytime sleepiness (EDS), as well as the impact of SDB on quality of life. Gottlieb et al. [15] reported an association not only between EDS and the AHI, but between sleepiness and snoring alone. This study also suggested that as much as half the middle-aged adult population may have levels of SDB that are associated with excessive sleepiness. Thus, SDB may contribute substantially to the population burden of excessive sleepiness, an important cause of accidents, impaired social performance, and reduced quality of life. Because the elderly have additional causes of EDS, the superimposition of SDB in this population would be expected to have an even more profound impact on the health status and quality of life of the aged. Baldwin and colleagues [16] demonstrated that SDB is associated with impaired quality of life equivalent to other chronic diseases in the general US population.

The SHHS has also provided important information regarding the diagnosis of SDB. In a study by Young et al., male gender, age, BMI, neck girth, snoring, and repeated breathing pauses were independent correlates of significant SDB. Moreover, as age increased, the magnitude of associations for SDB and body habitus, snoring, and breathing pauses decreased [17]. This finding indicates that SDB is more likely to go undiagnosed in the elderly. A better understanding of predictive factors for SDB in older adults is therefore needed.

Finally, data from the SHHS suggest a clear lessening in quantity and quality of sleep with age as determined by total sleep time (TST), sleep efficiency, and arousal index. This decline appears to be more rapid in males compared with that in females [18].

5.3 Polysomnography

5.3.1 History and Background

A sleep study or nocturnal PSG involves the recording of multiple physiologic parameters relevant to sleep. Both PSG and the practice of sleep medicine originated in the late 1950s and have evolved together since that time. Their beginnings were precipitated by the discovery and investigation of rapid eye movement (REM) sleep and sleep apnea.

Kleitman and Aserinsky [19] discovered REM sleep, and their findings appeared in their seminal paper published in 1953. However, it was not until Dement and Klietman [20] quantified and further characterized REM sleep in the late 1950s that the first all-night sleep recordings were performed. With the independent discovery of sleep apnea in the early 1960s by Gastaut et al. [21] from France and Jung and Kuhlo [22] from Germany, respiratory and cardiac sensors became a routine component of all-night sleep recordings. In 1974, Jerome Holland, a member of the Stanford University Sleep Disorders Clinic, coined the term PSG to refer to the entire constellation of physiologic variables measured during an all-night sleep study [23].

5.3.2 Fundamental Principles [24]

Routine PSG serves three primary functions: monitoring, staging and characterizing sleep, detecting SDB and its consequences, and documenting and quantifying periodic limb movements during sleep (PLMS). PSG can also diagnose parasomnias (abnormal nocturnal behaviors). Examples of parasomnias include sleep walking, REM sleep behavior disorder, and nocturnal seizures. Special montages may be required for the evaluation of nocturnal seizures (Figure 5.2).

The electroencephalogram (EEG) is the core measurement of PSG. The four stages of non-REM (NREM) sleep (stages 1, 2, 3, 4) are distinguished from each other principally by their specific EEG characteristics. The EEG will also detect arousals or awakenings from sleep. The most common locations of head electrodes for recording the EEG during sleep are C3 (left central), C4 (right central), O1 (left occipital) and O2 (right occipital). Head electrodes are typically referenced to another electrode that is usually placed on the contralateral mastoid or ear lobe. It is recommended that either C3/A2 or C4/A1 be used to assess sleep stages, where A2 refers to the right auricular and A1 to the left auricular lead, respectively (Figure 5.3).

In addition to monitoring the EEG, staging REM sleep also requires the measurement of bilateral eye movements, the cardinal sign of REM sleep, and chin muscle activity. Phasic bursts of REMs are measured by electrodes placed at the right outer canthus (ROC) and left outer canthus (LOC). Electrodes are placed over the mentalis/SUBMENTALIS muscles to monitor chin electromyogram (EMG).

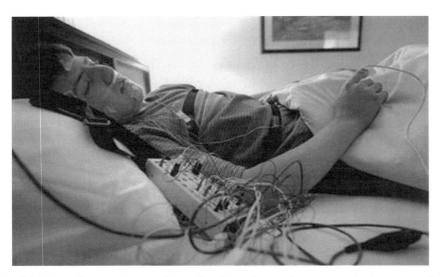

Fig. 5.2 Picture demonstrating a patient undergoing a sleep study or nocturnal polysomnography with the "typical" devices and monitors attached (Image Credit: Newsweek Health, Issue: March 3, 2005)

Fig. 5.3 Placement of
standard
electroencephalogram (EEG)
electrodes for conventional
polysomnography

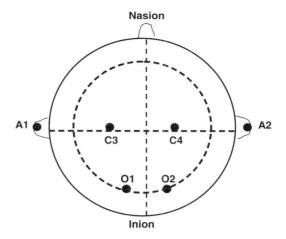

Monitoring tibialis anterior EMG permits the detection of PLMS, which can cause EEG arousals and consequent sleep fragmentation (Figure 5.4).

Staging of sleep permits the clinician to calculate and quantify numerous indices that can assist in the evaluation of sleep disorders such as circadian rhythm abnormalities and insomnia. These variables include sleep latency (SL; time it takes to fall asleep after lights out), REM latency (time it takes to reach the first REM period), TST, sleep efficiency [TST divided by time in bed (TIB)], number of transient arousals and awakenings, number of sleep stage changes, percentage of total NREM sleep as well as the individual NREM sleep stages, percentage of REM sleep, and intrusion of alpha activity into deeper sleep.

SDB is detected by monitoring airflow and respiratory effort. Methods to monitor airflow include pneumotachography, which typically measures airflow; nasal airway pressure; thermistors and thermocouples, which measure changes in temperature; and expired carbon dioxide sensing. The most common technique for assessing respiratory effort is the measurement of rib cage and abdominal movement. Methods to measure respiratory movement include strain gauges, inductance plethysmography, and impedance pneumography. Additional techniques to monitor respiratory effort include intercostal EMGs, measuring changes in pleural pressure with an esophageal balloon, a static charge-sensitive bed, and digital video.

An obstructive respiratory event is diagnosed when there is a significant decrease in airflow associated with continued respiratory effort. A central respiratory event is scored when the diminished airflow occurs in the setting of no respiratory effort. Although their definition is somewhat controversial, an apnea is typically defined as complete or near complete ($<25\%$ of "baseline" breathing) cessation of airflow, lasting ≥ 10 s [25, 26]. A hypopnea is defined as a decrease in airflow to $<70\%$ but $>25\%$ of the amplitude of "baseline" breathing for ≥ 10 s and associated either with an oxyhemoglobin desaturation of ≥ 3 or 4% or an arousal from sleep characterized by alpha activity or EEG speeding [25, 26]. To diagnose a hypopnea, Medicare requires an oxyhemoglobin desaturation of $\geq 4\%$ [27]. A respiratory effort-related

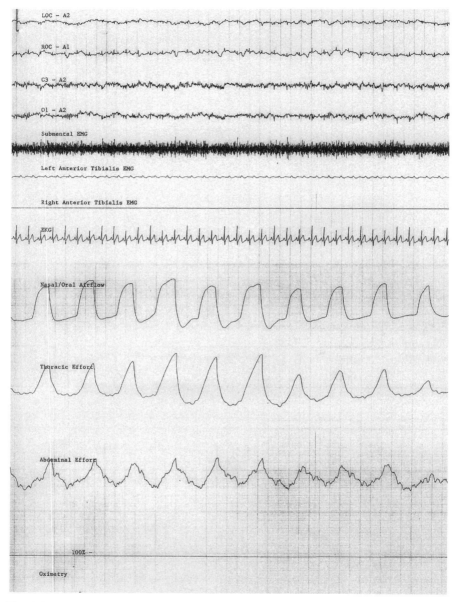

Fig. 5.4 Typical physiologic parameters measured and signals generated during conventional polysomnography. LOC-A1 and ROC-A2 monitor extraocular movements, which are important for identifying rapid eye movement (REM) sleep. LOC = left outer canthus; ROC = right outer canthus; nasion = nose; A1 = left auricular; A2 = right auricular; C3 = left central; C4 = right central; O1 = left occipital; O2 = right occipital

arousal (RERA) is scored when an obstructive respiratory event is terminated by an arousal from sleep but does not meet criteria for either an apnea or a hypopnea [28, 29] (Figure 5.5).

The usual physiologic consequences of SDB that are measured during PSG are arterial oxyhemoglobin saturation (SaO_2) with pulse oximetry, and cardiac arrhythmias and ischemia with an electrocardiogram (ECG). The EEG detects arousals or awakenings from sleep caused by abnormal breathing events. One can also monitor transcutaneous carbon dioxide, blood pressure, and autonomic nervous system arousal.

The severity of SDB is often based on the AHI, which is the number of apneas plus hypopneas per hour of sleep. The respiratory disturbance index (RDI) is another marker of disease severity and is the number of apneas plus hypopneas plus RERAs per hour of sleep [28, 29]. A normal AHI and RDI are <5 [28, 29]. A normal AHI with a RDI ≥5 is consistent with the diagnosis of upper airway resistance syndrome (UARS) [28, 29]. With this disorder, abnormal obstructive breathing events cause arousals from sleep and consequent EDS without causing an apnea or hypopnea or oxygen desaturation.

According to the American Academy of Sleep Medicine (AASM), diagnostic criteria for the OSA-hypopnea syndrome (OSAHS) include [29]:

1. An AHI or RDI ≥5 *plus*
2. EDS that is not better explained by other factors *or*
3. Two or more of the following (not better explained by other factors)
    a. Choking or gasping during sleep
    b. Recurrent awakenings during sleep
    c. Unrefreshing sleep
    d. Daytime fatigue
    e. Impaired concentration

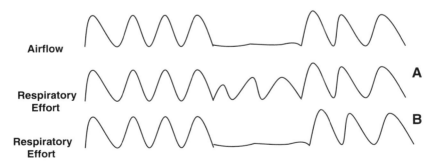

Fig. 5.5 Comparison of obstructive (A) versus central (B) apnea. Both events are associated with complete or near complete cessation of airflow. An obstructive apnea (A) is associated with no airflow despite continued respiratory effort. With a central apnea (B), the lack of airflow is secondary to the absence of respiratory effort from failure of the respiratory center in the medulla to stimulate the respiratory muscles

For the Centers for Medicare and Medicaid Services to reimburse nasal CPAP treatment for OSAHS, the following criteria must be fulfilled [27]:

1. AHI >15 *or*
2. AHI >5 with any of the following: hypertension, stroke, sleepiness, ischemic heart disease, insomnia, or mood disorders

The severity of SDB can be defined using a clinical dimension, i.e., sleepiness or the AHI. One classification schema defines mild OSAHS as an AHI of 5–15; an AHI of 15–30 is indicative of moderate disease; and an AHI >30 is consistent with severe OSAHS [28, 29].

A multiple sleep latency test (MSLT) is a series of four to six nap opportunities beginning approximately 2 h after morning awakening [30]. It is usually performed after a nocturnal PSG. The naps are performed at 2-h intervals; patients are tested under standardized conditions. SL and whether REM sleep occurs during the nap are recorded. The sleep latencies are then averaged to provide a mean SL.

5.3.3 Clinical Use and Application

The major role of nocturnal PSG is in the diagnosis of the patient with EDS. SDB and PLMS are the major disorders that can be diagnosed with PSG, although the actual role of PLMS as a cause of EDS is unclear. Because a single, brief clinical observation alone is an ineffective screening or diagnostic procedure for detecting the presence or determining the severity of SDB, nocturnal PSG is required if sleep apnea is suspected [31]. Nap studies performed during the day to diagnose SDB have approximately 75% diagnostic sensitivity at best [32]. The reason for this is that REM sleep, the most vulnerable sleep stage for the development of obstructive SDB because of the loss of upper airway muscle tone, infrequently occurs in naps. Consequently, a negative nap study must be followed by a nocturnal PSG. Thus, if after a thorough evaluation no clear cause of EDS is identified (i.e., insufficient sleep, shift work sleep disorder, medications), or SDB is suspected clinically, performing a nocturnal PSG is a reasonable next step. If the nocturnal PSG does not establish a cause of EDS, performing an MSLT the following morning is reasonable. An MSLT will help establish the diagnosis of narcolepsy and idiopathic hypersomnia, two other causes of EDS.

Because of the expense, the fact that at most one or two nights of data are obtained, the increased night-to-night variability of sleep typically seen with insomnia, and the fact that laboratory sleep may not be an accurate representation of the patient's sleep in the home, the AASM does not recommend nocturnal PSG as a first-line diagnostic tool in the assessment of chronic insomnia [33]. Nocturnal PSGs are also not recommended for the routine evaluation of patients with circadian rhythm abnormalities such as shift work sleep disorder [33]. While cardiorespiratory disorders such as chronic obstructive pulmonary disease and congestive heart failure can be associated nocturnal hypoxemia, nocturnal oximetry alone usually suffices. A nocturnal PSG is indicated in the setting of cardiopulmonary diseases only if there is a clinical suspicion of obstructive or central sleep apnea [33]. Of course, a nocturnal PSG may be considered later in any of these circumstances, after other avenues of investigation and treatment have been unyielding or ineffective.

If the history and other characteristics are highly suggestive and typical of the diagnosis, a nocturnal PSG is not indicated for the routine investigation of parasomnias [33]. However, PSG becomes important if there are atypical features such as age of onset or when the behaviors occur during the sleep cycle; if the behaviors are potentially injurious to the patient or others, or seriously disturb the patient's home life; if the behaviors are repetitive and stereotypical, which suggests the possibility of nocturnal seizures; when EDS is present; or when there are forensic concerns [33].

The MSLT provides an objective measure of sleepiness and is indicated as part of the evaluation of suspected narcolepsy and idiopathic hypersomnia [33].

5.3.4 Usage in the Home

At the present time, the "gold standard" for diagnosing sleep apnea and other sleep disorders is standard attended PSG performed by a technician in a sleep laboratory. However, the rapid increase in referrals for standard, in-laboratory PSG has prompted the development of portable monitors that can potentially be used in the patient's home. In 1992, the AASM, formerly the American Sleep Disorders Association (ASDA), classified portable monitors into four types or levels [34]. Although the bioparameters recorded by level II, III, and IV devices depend on the manufacturer and user-defined protocols, Table 5.1 portrays the typical montages utilized.

Table 5.1 Sensor Modalities Recorded by Different Levels of Devices

Parameter	Level I	Level II	Level III[a]	Level IV[a,b]
EEG	+	+	−	−
EOG	+	+	−	−
EMG Submentalis (chin)	+	+	−	−
ECG	+	+	+	−
Airflow	+	+	+	−
Respiratory effort	+	+	+	−
SaO2	+	+	+	+
Body position	+	Optional	Optional	−
EMG Anterior tibialis	+	+	−	−
Attended	+	−	−	−

EEG, electroencephalogram; EOG, electrooculogram; EMG, electromyogram;
ECG, electrocardiogram; SaO$_2$, oxygen saturation.
[a] These are typical montages; others exist.
[b] Single or dual; examples include adding snoring or airflow.

Theoretical advantages of home studies include that patients may sleep better, that they may prefer to be studied at home, that recordings at home will more accurately reflect the patient's "usual" sleep, more rapid diagnosis, and treatment if there is a delay in obtaining an in-laboratory PSG, and cost. Theoretical disadvantages of unattended home studies include the absence of observational information and support from a technician, and unnoticed sensor failure or inaccuracy. Data loss rates of 20% have been reported for level II studies [35]. In addition, two studies found that patients preferred in-laboratory PSG to a level II portable monitor, possibly because of patient concerns about safety or equipment failure [35, 36]. Theoretical disadvantages of level III and IV studies, which do not monitor sleep or PLMS, include not knowing if the patient slept or if REM sleep occurred, which can result in an underestimation of the severity of SDB; the inability to accurately calculate an AHI or RDI, which may also diminish sensitivity; the inability to detect other causes of EDS such as the UARS and PLMS.

In 2003, an evidence-based medicine review of the literature concerning portable monitoring for diagnosing SDB was compiled and published. From this review, which was a joint effort by the AASM, the American Thoracic Society, and the American College of Chest Physicians, practice parameters were formulated [37]. On the basis of the present evidence, it was concluded that only level III devices attended by a qualified technologist can reliably determine whether a patient has an AHI greater than 15 events per hour of recording time [37]. There was insufficient evidence to recommend attended or unattended level II devices, unattended level III devices, and attended or unattended level IV devices [37].

One efficient and potentially cost-effective approach to diagnosing SDB is to conduct a split-night, diagnostic pressure titration study. With this approach, which is the one we employ, the first 2 h of an in-laboratory PSG are spent evaluating for the presence of SDB. If the AHI is greater than 15, the remainder of the night is spent determining the optimal nasal CPAP. This approach is acceptable for about 80% of patients [38]. Because a positive home study requires subsequent nasal CPAP titration, such an approach saves money by avoiding the cost of a home study. Performing a home study will result in savings only if SDB is not severe enough to have been split on an in-laboratory study, but severe enough to have been diagnosed by a home study. On the basis of the recent evidence-based recommendations, if a home device is chosen, it should be an attended level III study.

5.4 Actigraphy

5.4.1 History and Background

Often when we picture a bad night's sleep, we envision someone who is restless, tossing, and turning while trying everything they can to go to sleep. Although this can be true more often than not for those with trouble sleeping, everyone has a degree of restlessness that affects the quality and restorative nature of their sleep.

These movements during sleep were not objectively measured until 1922 by J.S. Szymansky. Since then, many different types of equipment have been used to monitor movement during sleep ranging from photography and video cameras to EEG movement artifacts [39]. Tryon [40] has compiled a comprehensive history of the development of activity monitoring in medicine and his effort will not be duplicated here.

As technological advances allowed for smaller components to be manufactured, devices designed to record limb movement, known as actigraphs, were developed. Kupfer et al. [41, 42] were the first to develop this new technology to study differences between sleep and wake states, while Colburn et al. [43] developed a similar device around the same time. These had some of the same aspects as current actigraphs such as being self-contained (i.e., not wired to a larger device) and having the ability to record data for later use [44]. However, these and others developed later [45–47] were analog-based models instead of the current digital models we see today. These digital models have taken advantage of microprocessors and ever shrinking component sizes to not only allow automatic scoring using computer algorithms but also to be packaged into a wristwatch-sized device [44].

5.4.2 Fundamental Principles

Current actigraphs are based on accelerometers that output different numeric values with respect to changes in orientation and the speed in which the change occurs. These values are sampled multiple times a second, aggregated over a set epoch (usually 1 min), and stored locally on the device for later retrieval. The aggregation of the data allows the actigraphs to record movements for many days in a row, providing longitudinal data about circadian rhythms and the individual's activity patterns [39]. The original analog actigraphs' data had to be manually scored in a time-consuming process that has now been replaced by computer algorithms in digital actigraphs (Figure 5.6).

Three basic methods have been used as the backbones of these algorithms. The first, known as "time above threshold," simply assesses the time per epoch that the numerical value of the accelerometer's output was above a set threshold. This failed to detect small movements while also failing to adequately describe the magnitude or speed of the movements. The second, known as the "zero-crossing method," logs the number of times the signal from the accelerometer crosses zero. This has similar drawbacks to the first method while also being susceptible to high-frequency signals being recorded as large amounts of movement. The third method, known as "digital integration" calculates the area under the curve of the accelerometer's output signal. This provides data missing from the first two but fails to provide the information about frequency and duration that the first two provide. Thus, a combination of more than one method, as used in some devices today, is probably the best method to accurately log the most information. One ongoing problem is the proliferation of algorithms, especially those that are device specific. This makes it hard to compare studies that are done with different devices [7].

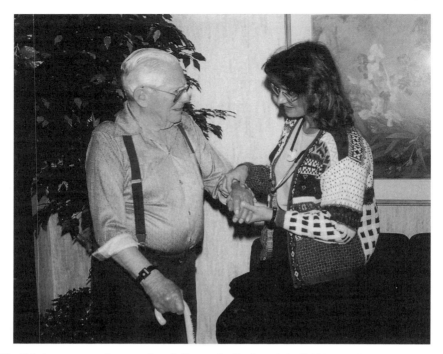

Fig. 5.6 A person wearing an actigraph (Image Credit: Copyright © 2007 Respironics/Minimitter. All rights reserved.)

Actigraphs can be placed on either the wrist or the ankle to monitor different limb movements. The non-dominant wrist tends to be the place of choice, although ankle movements can be especially important in monitoring periodic limb movement or restless leg syndrome. Placement is important because artifacts could be created if the subject constrains one of their limbs because of their sleeping position (i.e., sleeping on one side or placing their arm under the pillow). Non-compliance in wearing the actigraph can also cause artifacts of lack of movement that could be read as sleep or, on the contrary, movement artifacts can be caused if the subject is sleeping in a moving vehicle [7].

5.4.3 Clinical Use

Although the ASDA, now the AASM, does not recommend the use of actigraphy for diagnosis of sleep disorders, it did determine that they are a useful addition to subjective data, such as sleep diaries and other paper-based sleep assessment instruments, in examining multiple days of sleep–wake patterns. Having the ability to record many nights of data in addition to daytime activity provides useful information that cannot be obtained through PSG or subjective data. In fact, in disorders such as periodic limb movement where there is variability from night to night, actigraph could provide a clearer picture of the severity of the disorder [44].

5.4.4 Home Use

Actigraphy is mostly used outside the clinic. By having the ability to record weeks of data at a time, actigraphs have become very useful in providing objective, longitudinal data in the home environment. Despite some of the limitations mentioned earlier, the actigraph's ability to objectively detect minute movements during sleep, many of which are not perceived by the individual, allows it to be useful in assessing quality of sleep and indicators of common disorders such as insomnia, sleep apnea, periodic limb movement, and restless leg syndrome. When used properly in the home, actigraphy has an advantage over subjective assessment tools such as sleep diaries and logs or other survey-based instruments by being able to detect disturbances of which the subject is not aware. When data are collected over many nights, formulations about the circadian rhythms and sleep pattern behavior can be assessed objectively. This is useful both in helping determine effects of sleep disorders and also helping physicians assess the effectiveness of treatments they prescribe for the patients. However, actigraphy in the home remains far from being a diagnostic tool on its own because it only examines activity and has limitations in an unattended setting [48].

5.4.5 Applications

One of the main applications of actigraphy is in studies of the circadian rhythms. The human rest–activity cycle is accurately portrayed by actigraphs, and their data are quite useful in determining changes in sleep patterns and behavior that may require treatment. In addition, the effects of this treatment can be analyzed using actigraphy to detect any changes once the treatment is started. This objective outcome analysis is important in evaluating new ways to treat circadian rhythm-based sleep disorders [48].

Because of the longitudinal nature of actigraphy data and its convenience to allow researchers to conduct studies in the subjects' homes, actigraphs are quite useful in assessing sleep in the elderly or other populations, including children and the homebound, where clinical visits might be too much of an adversity. Older adults are more susceptible to problems with their sleep, especially those related to circadian behavior [44]. Additionally, dementia is a significant problem in older adults. Actigraphy has been used in both populations to detect disruptions in the circadian rhythms as well as sleep fragmentation leading to a poor night's rest [44,48]. The interactions of older adults and their caregivers studied with actigraphy have revealed that activity levels of the two groups were different during the day whereas being closer at night. In addition, it was shown that it was the elder who often interrupted the sleep of the caregiver, rather than the caregiver checking on the older adult [48]. Actigraphy also makes it possible to objectively study nursing home and assisted living populations, for both memory care and non-memory care residents. These studies could lead to more information about the symptoms and causes of dementia in addition to a greater understanding of the sleep behavior of that population and how their sleep requirements might differ from people in other stages of life.

Overall, actigraphs provide the longitudinal information needed to assess circadian rhythm-based sleep disorders but still lack the necessary details to accurately diagnose many sleep disorders. Improvements in scoring algorithms with perhaps the addition of other technology, such as environmental, positional, and/or basic physiological sensors, might allow actigraphs to play a role in the diagnostic world and make it easier to assess sleep in the home environment.

5.5 Ballistocardiography

5.5.1 History and Background

J.W. Gordon observed more than just his weight every time he stepped onto a spring scale back in the latter part of the 19th century. While he was standing on the scale, he noticed that the needle would fluctuate in conjunction with his heartbeat. Before this, as early as 1786, movements of the body similar to these had been observed in a case of hyperthyroidism, as these body movements are greatly exaggerated in this condition. In 1877, Gordon recorded similar movements from a bed he designed, but from a healthy person. This bed was suspended from the ceiling and the signal was traced on a smoked drum through the use of mechanical levers. And, thus, the field of ballistocardiography (BCG) was born [49] (Figure 5.7).

Twenty-six years later, in 1905, Yandell Henderson made a similar observation to Gordon's about the spring scale, unaware of the previous work done, and constructed a similar bed. In 1913, Satterthwaite, like Henderson and Gordon, made a similar observation about the scale but was also uninformed of any previous work. He made some records by extending the tip of the scale. Nine years later, Heald and Tucker were the first people to observe and identify normal respiratory variation. In 1928, Angenheister, a geophysicist, noted that his seismograph would produce fluctuations when he placed it next to a patient lying on a rigid surface [49].

In 1936, Isaac Starr [50], known by many as the father of BCG, was in search of a non-invasive method to improve on the established study of cardiac function. Upon meeting Henderson at a program held by the Circulation Section of the American Physiological Society geared toward studying cardiac function, Starr decided to pursue Henderson's principles while taking advantage of new technologies such as optical magnification. By adding springs to Henderson's design while making additional structural improvements, Starr was able to obtain ballistocardiogram waveforms with reasonable amplitude and without the interference of respiration [49].

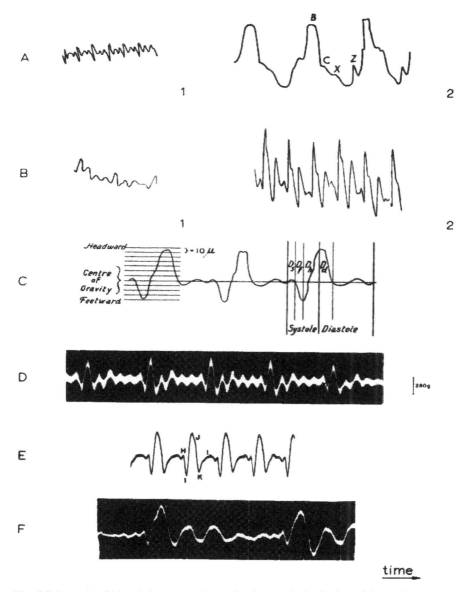

Fig. 5.7 Records of historic interest and records taken at the beginning of the modern era. A: Gordon's original records (1877). Subject standing on scale (1) and lying on a bed suspended by four ropes (2). B: Landois' records of subjects standing upright (1880); (1) normal, (2) of a case of aortic regurgitation. Time and amplitude ratios are the same as in Landois' figures. C: Henderson's record on a normal subject lying on a suspended table (1905). D: Record taken with Starr's original high-frequency instrument on a healthy subject lying (1939). E: A record taken by Nickerson's low-frequency instrument (1945) on a subject lying at rest. F: One of Dock's shin-bar records (1949) [49] (Image Credit: Used with permission from Lippincott, Williams and Wilkins, Inc.)

5.5.2 *Fundamental Principles*

In its most basic principle, the BCG is a recording of minute movements associated with cardiac contraction and relaxation as well as the movement of blood throughout the vasculature [51]. There are actually two different types of BCGs—one based on displacement and one based on force. The displacement BCG, also known as the ultra low frequency (ULF) BCG usually involves an apparatus that isolates the patient from the floor. This isolation is usually done either with torsion springs and linkages or by floating the patient on a thin layer of a low friction material, typically air [52]. The internal force resulting from the energy generated by contracting internal body organs would produce displacements that can be recorded [53]. Velocity and acceleration waveforms can also be obtained by taking a simple derivative and second derivative of the displacement waveform, respectively. The waveform itself is mostly characterized by how strong a force is generated by the ventricles and the material properties of the arterial system, largely compliance. Figure 5.8 [54] provides a clear correspondence of how a ULF BCG waveform corresponds to measurements that are currently accepted as clinical standards. Specifically the slope and amplitude of the HIJ complex corresponds to the mechanical forces that are a result of the QRS electrical impulse caused by the depolarization of the left ventricle. The LMN complex corresponds to the mechanical forces that are a result of the T-wave, which occurs before the aortic valve closing. Thus, HIJ is associated with systole

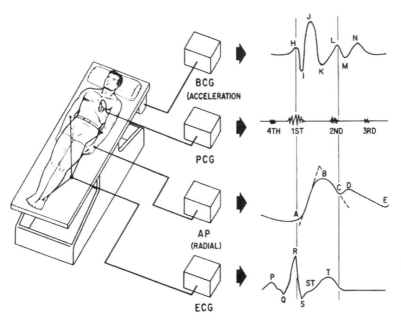

Fig. 5.8 ULF BCG Correspondence to common cardiac measurements [54] (Image Credit: Used with permission from S. Karger AG)

and LMN is associated with diastole. The lettering convention is the standard set by the American Heart Association's Committee on Ballistocardiographic Terminology [55].

The BCG based on force, also known as the high-frequency (HF) BCG, uses similar, but slightly different conventions as compared with the ULF BCG. Rather than looking at the displacement from the internal force generated by blood flow, these BCGs are focused on the force characteristics themselves. To obtain this information, the body is rigidly supported rather than mounted on a near-frictionless surface [56]. Six different possible forces can be recorded (head-to-foot, side-to-side, front-to-back, along with three associated moments), although the strongest force is the head-to-foot. Additionally, this waveform can also be obtained from a seated subject in addition to a supine one. Figure 5.9 presents a simplified model representing the HF BCG, together with a piezoelectric force transducer [56].

This figure represents the body as having an outer rigid part (m_b) and an inner compliant part (c) while the heart is a rigid mass (m_h). The mass of the seat platform (m_s) is also rigid and the piezoelectric sensor is represented as a spring with compliance (c_q). The internal acting force, primarily from the movement of blood in the system, is translated to the platform, displacing the attached sensor [56]. Similar to the ULF BCG as seen in Figure 5.10 [55], the HIJK complex represents the systolic while the MN represents the diastolic forces. The major difference is the addition of the K portion and the lack of the L portion [55].

5.5.3 Initial Clinical Use

Upon clinical application of the BCG, research in the field was accelerated and new techniques for acquisition and analysis were invented. From the 1950s to the 1970s,

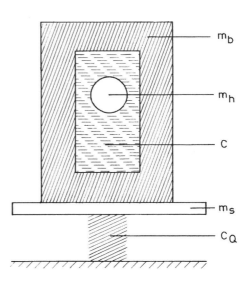

Fig. 5.9 Model of an HF BCG acquisition system [56] (Image Credit: Used with permission from S. Karger AG)

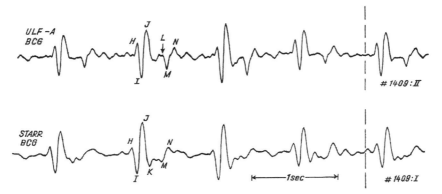

Fig. 5.10 Typical ULF & HF (Starr) BCG Waveforms with standard labels [55] (Image Credit: Used with permission from S. Karger AG)

much knowledge was gained. For example, Starr showed that initial cardiac forces correlate to life duration and susceptibility to ischemic heart disease. Additionally, it was shown that the average force generated by the BCG were reduced as a person aged [50]. Unfortunately, high expectations and hopes for this new technology simply resulted in disappointments because of a lack of adequate analysis tools [57]. In addition, the ECG quickly usurped this technology as a more practical way to measure cardiac function.

5.5.4 Current Use and Applications

Technological advancements during the latter part of the 20th century have allowed BCG to become practical and could open doors to provide additional key information about cardiopulmonary function. Because of the emergence and standardization of the ECG, the current focus of BCG-based research has moved toward comprehensive sleep analysis, rather than just measuring cardiac function. New technology based on the BCG still involves unconstrained monitoring of cardiac function, generally using the force-based version of the BCG, but it also includes the ability to record forces from respiratory effort and gross movement. These technological advances have contributed to making BCG hardware portable and usable in the home environment, where sensors can be placed in a bed without interfering with a person's sleep. Comprehensive objective data that can be acquired without altering a person's sleep are critical to understanding sleep disorders and aspects of sleep such as quality and day-to-day patterns. Being able to study sleep in a person's home environment for long periods of time could lead to breakthroughs in diagnosis and treatment of sleep disorders. Additionally, longitudinal monitoring of sleep patterns and sleep quality could lead to better overall management of chronic disease conditions and general improvement in quality of life.

The applications of this type of technology are numerous. In addition to potentially diagnosing and screening for sleep disorders, efficacy of treatments such as

CPAP or medication could be objectively evaluated. Additionally, in assisted living and skilled nursing environments, the technology could provide professional care-givers with information about the residents' sleep quality, allowing them to make the necessary adjustments to aspects of care, such as pain management and environmental control, to improve the residents' quality of life. In a hospital setting, movement could be monitored to reduce the risk for the development of pressure sores while also being able to alert nurses as to when patients are awaking from anesthesia after surgery. As the technology becomes more portable, it can also be adapted to fit into wheelchairs to assess pressure sore risk while also providing non-critical physiological monitoring.

5.6 Portable PSG Devices

5.6.1 Level II PSG

One of the better studied level II systems is the Compumedics portable PS-2 monitoring system (Abbottsville, Australia). It is the home system that was utilized in the SHHS. The usual recording montage of the PS-2 system includes C3/A1; C4/A2 EEG; bilateral EOGs; a bipolar submental EMG; thoracic and abdominal excursions, as detected by inductance plethysmography; airflow, as detected by oronasal thermocouple (Protec, Woodinville, WA, USA); SaO_2, as detected by finger pulse oximetry (Nonin, Minneapolis, MN, USA), ECG, body position, as detected by a mercury gauge sensor; and ambient light by a light sensor secured to the recording garment; right and left leg movements can be monitored with piezoelectric cells. The data recorded are then downloaded to the Compumedics PS-Series Sleep System to enable the study to be analyzed using the Compumedics software.

In a recent comparison between unattended home versus attended in-laboratory studies using the Compumedics PS-2 system, the authors demonstrated that there was no difference in median RDI in the 64 individuals studied [58]. This finding persisted despite using multiple definitions of the RDI. However, across the range of RDIs in this study, there was a small biphasic effect on the difference between the laboratory and home setting. At mean RDIs >20, the laboratory RDI was consistently greater; at mean RDIs <20, the home RDI was greater. These differences in RDI between settings resulted in a rate of disease mis-classification of 6–25%. The authors indicated that this rate is similar to that expected from night to night variation for studies performed on different evenings at the same location [59]. These differences were not secondary to quality of recording, age, sex, or body mass index. The study also found that median values for arousal index were similar between the home and the in-laboratory studies. However, the laboratory setting was associated with a shorter sleep time, poorer sleep efficiency, and a very small but significant increase in stage 1 sleep and decrease in REM sleep. Currently, and until additional and larger studies are performed, level II PSG should not replace in-laboratory level 1 studies.

5.6.2 Level III Studies

5.6.2.1 SNAP [60–62]

The SNAP Laboratories LLC sleep diagnostic system (Wheeling, IL, USA) consists of a digital recorder with a removable Zip disc that can record up to 338 min of sleep time. Sensors record oronasal thermistor to detect airflow, oronasal sound, pulse oximetry, heart rate, and respiratory effort with a chest belt. Leg motion and body position can also be recorded. Digital data are then transferred to the SNAP system, where automatic processing is performed.

In an in-laboratory study of 60 subjects by Su et al., for an RDI ≥15, the SNAP device had a sensitivity of 83.9%, a negative predictive value (NPV) of 81.5%, a specificity of 75.9%, and a positive predictive value (PPV) of 78.8%. It correctly classified 80% of patients. In another in-laboratory study of 39 patients by Liesching et al., the severity of sleep apnea was misclassified by SNAP in approximately 65% of patients. This study's NPV was 13% and PPV 77%. Thus, basing clinical decisions on results from the SNAP device has the potential risk of missing the diagnosis of OSA up to 20% of the time. Moreover, the PPV of the SNAP system requires that a positive study be confirmed. Another problem is the "black box" nature of the scoring of respiratory events. Because the scoring software is proprietary, the interpreter never sees the raw data. Finally, the in-laboratory data of this and other studies with the SNAP system requires confirmation in the unattended home setting.

5.6.2.2 POLY-MESAM [63]

The POLY-MESAM (PM) device is an upgrade from its predecessor, the MESAM-4. It consists of a monitor with seven channels: (1) a joint nasal and oral thermister to determine airflow, (2) a laryngeal microphone, (3) a 3-channel ECG, (4) a thoracic and (5) abdominal stress-sensitive belt to determine respiratory effort, (6) a body position sensor and (7) a pulse oximeter. The accompanying computer software calculates the AHI, apnea index (AI), hypopnea index (HI), oxygen desaturation index (ODI), heart rate variation index (HRVI), and movement index. The ODI is the number of desaturation events per hour of recording.

Verse et al. performed an in-laboratory study of the PM device on 53 patients. Although there was a high degree of correlation between the findings of the level III and level I studies, in general, the level III device underestimated the severity of sleep apnea. Moreover, this underestimation increased with increasing severity of disease. Although the sensitivity for detecting an AHI >10 was 92%, it was 71.4% for an AHI >20. At least one explanation for this discrepancy is that the PM device, because it does not stage sleep, employs TIB rather than TST to determine its indices. The results of this study indicate that up to 20% of OSA patients were not recognized by the PM unit. In contrast, the specificity was reasonable, at approximately 96–97%. Once again, the PM unit, like the SNAP device, requires confirmation in the unattended home setting.

5.6.3 Level IV Studies

5.6.3.1 Nocturnal (overnight) Pulse Oximetry [28]

Pulse oximeters determine arterial oxygen saturation (SaO_2) using spectrophoto-electrical techniques. A two-wavelength light transmitter and a receiver are placed on either side of a pulsating arterial vascular bed, usually on a digit, ear, or nasal site. The amplitude of the light detected by the receiver depends on the magnitude of the change in arterial pulse, the wavelengths transmitted through the arterial vascular bed, and the SaO_2. The underlying principles of pulse oximetry are that oxygenated and deoxygenated hemoglobins have different light absorptive properties and that these devices are sensitive only to tissues that pulsate. Therefore, theoretically, venous blood, connective tissue, skin pigment, and bone do not interfere with the measurement of SaO_2. Although all pulse eximeters are based on similar technology, they have different response characteristics that depend on the manufacturer, the sampling rate, the technology minimizing motion artifact, and the sensor location.

Overall, the consensus of the medical literature is that overnight pulse oximetry is a sensitive but not specific technique for identifying moderate to severe sleep apnea. Unfortunately, this device may miss up to 61% of patients with treatable sleep disorders such as mild sleep apnea, UARS, and PLMS [64]. However, results vary significantly from study to study, depending on the diagnostic criteria utilized for an abnormal oximetry result as well as for sleep apnea. For instance, in a study by Ebstein et al., a "deep" pattern (>4% desaturation to below 90% SaO_2) had a sensitivity of 73.6% and a specificity of 89.4% for diagnosing sleep apnea [64]. In contrast, a "fluctuating" pattern (either large desaturations or low-amplitude periodic desaturations without a minimum saturation level) was more sensitive (96.2%) but less specific (55.3%) [64]. Other studies have utilized an ODI threshold to define SDB. When a desaturation event was defined as a 2% decrease in SaO_2 from baseline and sleep apnea defined as an AHI > 15/h, Hussain et al. [65] noted that 40% of patients with SDB had a normal nocturnal pulse oximetry. Chiner et al. [66] reported that while an ODI ≥5 had a sensitivity of 82% and a specificity of 62% in diagnosing SDB, an ODI of ≥15 increased the specificity to 93%, but at the expense of decreasing sensitivity to 62%. Nineteen percent of patients in this study would have been "unclassified." Because of its poor diagnostic accuracy, nocturnal pulse oximetry is not cost effective in the diagnosis of SDB.

5.6.3.2 SNORESAT [67]

In an attempt to improve the accuracy of nocturnal pulse oximetry in the diagnosis of SDB, Issa and colleagues added a device that digitally recorded sound from a transducer applied to the chest. In this study of 129 patients, a snoring event was defined as a moving time average of sound that exceeded a threshold voltage level for greater than 0.26 s. A respiratory event was defined as a period of absent snoring for 10–120 s separating two snoring events, and associated with a decrease in

$SaO_2 > 3\%$. All data were stored and analyzed using a computer algorithm, which calculated the number of respiratory events per hour of recording mean apnea duration, mean lowest SaO_2, and number of desaturations $>3\%$. For detecting an RDI ≥ 7, the sensitivity of the SNORESAT device was 84% and the specificity 95%; for an RDI ≥ 20, the sensitivity and specificity were 90 and 98%, respectively. Again, this study was performed in a laboratory and requires verification in the unattended home setting.

5.7 Actigraphy Technology

Several companies produce actigraph technology. This has led to a proliferation of different hardware and algorithms making it difficult to determine which devices are the best for clinical use. Two of the more widely used actigraph brands are Ambulatory Monitoring's Motionlogger® and Mini-Mitter/Respironics' Actiwatch®. The overall basic principles of actigraphy have already been described earlier in the general section on actigraphy, so the focus here is to introduce currently

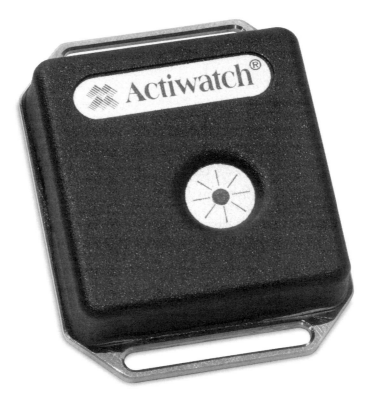

Fig. 5.11 MiniMitter Actiwatch (Image Credit: Copyright © 2007 Respironics/Minimitter. All rights reserved.)

available actigraph technology. Both of these aforementioned devices employ similar accelerometer-based sensors as their core data-acquisition tools and offer add-ons that provide additional data including light levels, ambient temperature, sound levels, data input by the user, and others. They both require an additional piece of hardware to transfer the data from the units themselves to the computer for analysis. Ambulatory Monitoring's software (Action W-2) is based on validated algorithms (Cole-Kripke, Sadeh, UCSD). Mini-Mitter/Respironics software (Actiware-Sleep 5.0) is based on another validated algorithm (Oakley) and has also been validated for use with insomnia patients (Lichstein) with the exception of the SL measures. Each of the devices samples the movement data several times a second before aggregating it into epoch lengths of only a few seconds or as long as a few minutes. Some of the devices have a fixed 1-min interval, at which they can store several days of data without information being downloaded to the computer. Ambulatory Monitoring's Basic Motionlogger has 2 MB of memory whereas Mini-Mitter/Respironics' Actiwatch-64 only has 64 KB of memory, so the Motionlogger can record data for longer periods of time [68, 69] (Figures 5.11 and 5.12).

In a direct comparison [70] of Ambulatory Monitoring's Basic Mini-Motionlogger and Mini-Mitter/Respironics' Actiwatch-L conducted by researchers at the Veterans Affairs Palo Alto Health Care System and Stanford University, 20 subjects were monitored while wearing both devices simultaneously. Each subject was studied for two non-consecutive nights and basic sleep characteristics including SL, TST, wake

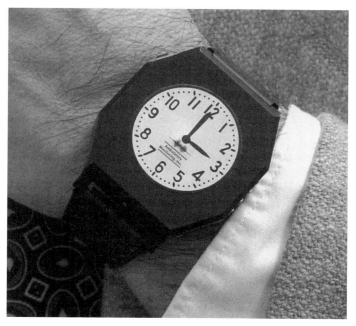

Fig. 5.12 Ambulatory Monitoring MotionLogger (Image Credit: Copyright © 2007 Ambulatory Monitoring, Inc. All rights reserved.)

after sleep onset, and sleep efficiency were calculated using the devices' respective software. Because of the comparison, it was concluded that the Actiwatch-L® set at medium sensitivity to wake performed similarly to the Basic Motionlogger on its default settings. However, there was no clinical standard in place to determine either of the device's clinical accuracy, so the study just focused on the inter-device comparison [70]. More validation and comparison studies should be conducted to provide the best clinical data possible when using actigraphy.

Both companies offer additional software packages for analyzing specific sleep disorders such as periodic limb movement and circadian rhythm disorders and the ability to wear the actigraphs on either the wrists or the ankles depending on the needed application.

5.8 Portable Sleep Monitoring Technology

5.8.1 The Static Charge-Sensitive Bed

Developed in Finland at the University of Turku in the late 1970s and early 1980s by a team led by J. Alihanka and K. Vaahtoranta, the static charge-sensitive bed (SCSB) was designed to meet the need for a non-invasive and passive way to monitor movements during sleep. The SCSB is basically a giant capacitor that changes in charge based on electrostatic build up from a person's movements while in bed [71]. It employs two metal sheets, each about 0.1-mm thick, that sandwich a stiff wooden board covered on both sides by two plastic sheets that form the "active layers," which generate the static charges. This assembly is then encased in a conductive shield to isolate it from static charges built up from surroundings or fabric. The potential difference between the plates changes with electrostatic energy generated from the interactions of the two active layers each time a person moves in bed. The system is extremely sensitive and can even discern minute movements from ballistocardiographic forces [72] (Figure 5.13).

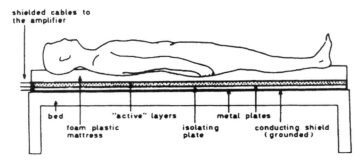

Fig. 5.13 Static Charge Sensitive Bed setup [72] (Image Credit: Used with permission from *American Journal of Physiology*)

Clearly, the SCSB has the ability to record physiological parameters without constraining the patient with wires or attached sensors, which is a limitation PSG-based sleep study. This inexpensive and simple approach also provides an option for recording important physiological characteristics during sleep longitudinally without affecting the person's comfort or environment, even enabling this type of study to be done at home [72]. However, the SCSB properties change based on the mattress used during the study and some physiological parameters are distorted when excessive movement is present [72]. The latter issue is normally not a problem during sleep, but could be a limitation for restless individuals. In addition, because it uses electrostatic energy, there is the risk of electrical shock, and that could limit the use of the SCSB for patients with pacemakers or other electrostatic sensitive devices.

The SCSB can be easily adapted for neonatal monitoring [73] in addition to being applicable to adult sleep studies. Differences in physiology have been observed during various sleep stages (72), which means that non-EEG sleep staging may be possible with the SCSB. Testing of SCSB-based sleep staging has been done by Jansen and Shankar with good results for sleep–wake determination, but this testing was only done on a few normal subjects [74], and would hence need to be confirmed in a larger study. Additionally, Polo has determined that the SCSB is a good screening tool for OSA, especially when combined with oximetry [51]. Further development of the SCSB for sleep analysis could provide an unconstrained method for conducting a sleep study in the home, which would be convenient for those in assisted living facilities and other eldercare settings who might not be able to undergo a PSG study at a clinic.

5.8.2 MESAM IV

The (MESAM) IV device was developed by a group led by Dr. Thomas Penzel at the Medical Poliklinik of Phillips-University Marburg in Germany back in the early 1990s [75, 76]. It specifically targeted the diagnosis of sleep-related breathing disorders. The MESAM IV is an ambulatory device that records heart rate through an ECG, snoring sounds using a laryngeal microphone, oxygen saturation with a conventional pulse oximeter, and body position by way of a sensor fixed to the sternum of the patient. These parameters all worked together to indirectly provide information about respiration. The data from the device can be scored either manually or automatically through the use of computer algorithms. Automatic analysis uses three separate indices to examine the likelihood of a respiratory event. These include (1) the HRVI, which counts the number of sudden increases in heart rate from baseline rest per hour, (2) the ODI, which counts the number of oxygen desaturations per hour that are over a 4% drop, and (3) the intermittent snoring index (ISI), which provides data about the snoring sound coming from the subject [77]. The manual method takes the heart rate, oxygen saturation, and snoring variables into account separately first, similar to the automatic method, but then checks for events that show variation in at least two of the variables. This method is more accurate than the automatic scoring method because it takes more than one variable into account [77].

The MESAM IV, using the manual scoring method in a controlled setting, is a helpful alternative to PSG when the subject is suspected to have OSA and it minimizes the amount of sensors attached to the subject. However, much further development will have to take place for it to become a clinically useful diagnostic tool; furthermore, the technology needs to be verified in an unattended setting.

5.8.3 Stanford University's SleepSmart^{TM} Bed Sheet

Designed by a team at Stanford University led by H.F. Machiel van der Loos, the SleepSmart^{TM} bed was developed to be a low-cost, multi-sensor sleep analysis tool. The system comprises a bed sheet that could detect heart rate, breathing rate, body movement, and temperature. It is based around two arrays of variable resistors, one force sensitive and the other temperature sensitive, that are arranged as seen in Fig. 5.14. The figure shows a concept for a prototype that layers the two arrays of sensors that produce various gradations of output displayed graphically and recorded for later use. By using a combination of analog signal processing and digital wavelet transformation, the heart rate and respiration signals can be extracted from the force sensitive resistors in addition to the movement data [78]. The force sensitive resistors were later replaced with a piezoelectric film, which provided better resolution for position and movement sensing [79].

The SleepSmart^{TM} system has the advantage of being an unconstrained monitor so the person is unaffected during sleep along with the fact that it can record

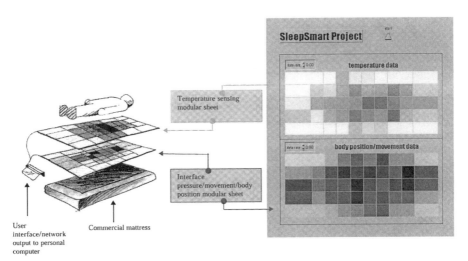

Fig. 5.14 SleepSmart^{TM} Bed Sheet Setup [78] (Image Credit: Used with permission from RESNA)

a rich dataset of physiological parameters. It can also estimate position based on moments from the movement force vectors. However, the device initially had difficulty obtaining a reasonably accurate heart rate signal and the sensor itself had to be close to the position of the heart (within 2 cm) [78] to even detect pulse. After a consulting firm conducted a feasibility study on the system, it was determined that the SleepSmart Bed Sheet was only capable of detecting breathing rate, body position, and movement while not being deemed feasible for entry into the medical market.

The piezoelectric film enables the sensor sheet to detect pressure points and would be quite applicable to detecting pressure sores as well as monitoring sleeping position. This combined with their other project called Morpheus, which is a robotic bed that can manipulate a person's position by adjusting in four different sections [80], may result with a system to automatically move people who are susceptible to positional sleep apnea or snoring, although much development must take place before it is clinically proven or commercially viable.

5.8.4 The Watch-PAT 100

Developed by Itamar Medical Limited in Caesarea, Israel, the Watch-PAT 100 primarily uses a physiological condition called peripheral arterial tone (PAT) to detect changes in characteristics such as autonomic nervous system activity and related vascular events [81]. It is able to achieve this by monitoring the changes in the volume of the fingertip influenced by vasoconstriction and dilation in addition to the changes in volume that result from pulsatile flow [82]. In combination with the optico-pneumatic sensor that detects the PAT signal, a pulse oximeter and actigraph are integrated into the wrist-worn device to provide additional information about oxygen desaturation and movement [83]. Itamar Medical's proprietary software is able to use the collected data to automatically calculate respiratory event indexes such as the AHI along with oxygen desaturation events and sleep, wake, and REM states [81]. It is FDA cleared and CE certified [82] (Figure 5.15).

The Watch-PAT 100 provides a non-invasive way to monitor physiological conditions by using a simple glove to which the sensors can be fitted in a comfortable manner so as to not disrupt sleep. It provides information on a similar, but less-detailed, level than PSG less expensively and more conveniently. In 2003, the Watch-PAT 100 was tested by researchers from the Harvard Medical School on 30 adult subjects [83]. They found a significant correlation ($r = 0.87$, $p < 0.001$) between the Watch-PAT 100 AHI and the PSG AHI, which was used as the gold standard in testing the device. Additionally, they found high sensitivity and specificity in classifying subjects based on specific thresholds of the AHI. However, the researchers found that the Watch-PAT 100 tended to overestimate those with low AHI and underestimate those with high AHI. The first could be related to movements and arousals that may occur from sleep fragmentation or other sleep disorders such as periodic limb movement. The second could be related to the density

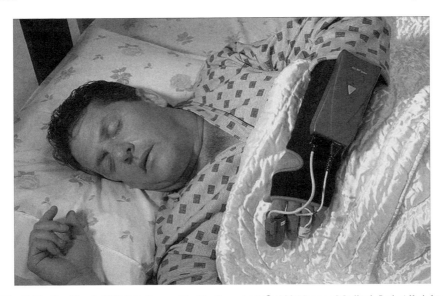

Fig. 5.15 The Watch-PAT 100 (Image Credit: Copyright © 2007 Itamar Medical, Ltd. All rights reserved.)

of events, resolution of the Watch-PAT 100, and its inability to detect such dense events. Additional testing outside the laboratory as well as further analysis on an event or epoch-by-epoch basis also needs to be done [83]. In 2006, 60 subjects were simultaneously monitored at the Technion-Israel Institute of Technology by the Watch-PAT 100 and polysomography recordings to determine the Watch-PAT's ability to detect REM sleep for people with various types of sleep apnea severity. Their sensitivity in correctly identifying epochs defined to be REM by polysomography analysis ranged from 65 to 76% whereas their specificity ranged from 93 to 95% [84].

With further development, the Watch-PAT 100 could become a useful tool for both screening and diagnosing sleep apnea that would make it more convenient to conduct home sleep assessments.

5.8.5 ARES Unicorder

The Apnea Risk Evaluation System (ARES) was recently developed by Advanced Brain Monitoring in Carlsbad, CA, USA, in conjunction with a questionnaire and software analysis package. Sleep studies with the ARES start first with a questionnaire (ARES Screener) that stratifies the patient's risk for having sleep apnea into three categories: none, low, or high. If from this questionnaire it is determined that a sleep study should be done, the ARES Unicorder is used to analyze the patient's sleep for up to four nights. It is a small device that is affixed to the forehead with a few peripheral sensors attached to the main box [85]. This device records important data including oxygen saturation, heart rate, snoring by way of a microphone, head position and movement through an accelerometer, and air flow through a nasal cannula. Their proprietary software (ARES Insight) uses the oximetry signal as the main indicator while using the other signals to help determine when arousals might be occurring. Their algorithm is based on the assumption that any desaturation followed by an arousal should be classified as a respiratory event. Arousals are marked by sharp changes in pulse, an increase in head movement, or snoring sounds following a desaturation [86]. The nasal airflow signal is used to detect any respiratory events where a desaturation might not be present and was only added recently after an initial study of the ARES device was done without it. The addition of the flow measurement capability improves the ability of the ARES system to detect respiratory events accurately removing the reliance on desaturation for event detection [87] (Figure 5.16).

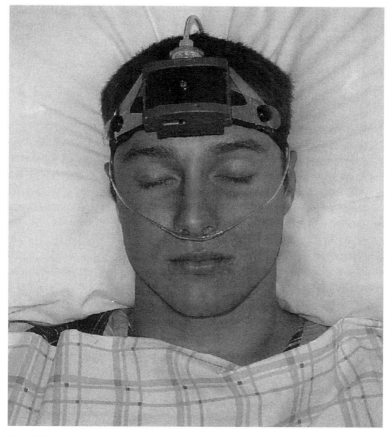

Fig. 5.16 ARES Unicorder (Image Credit: Copyright © 2007 Advanced Brain Monitoring, Inc. All rights reserved.)

The ARES system provides a convenient way to study sleep over multiple nights without the larger burden of PSG equipment or the need to come into the sleep laboratory. Its use of a nasal cannula may be inconvenient for some, but it provides a direct measurement of nasal airflow that can make detecting breathing stoppages easier than indirect methods of respiratory effort or reliance on desaturation. However, the ARES Unicorder consistently flags false-positive events that could lead to misdiagnosis of borderline or normal subjects, while still performing adequately for people with more severe sleep apnea.

The applications of the ARES system include its ability to bring the sleep apnea detection aspects of PSG into the home and record multiple nights of data in the subject's home environment. This ambulatory device is portable and can reach populations who might not be able to visit a sleep laboratory. Further development of the air flow sensor and ARES Insight algorithms could make the ARES an invaluable tool home assessment tool.

5.8.6 Sensewear Armband

Developed in 2001 by Body Media, Inc., in conjunction with the University of Pittsburgh Medical Center, the Sensewear® armband provides multi-sensor physiological and activity monitoring in the convenience of a wearable armband. Body Media's patented technology contains a skin temperature sensor, a galvanic skin response sensor that indirectly reflects the water content of the skin, and vasoconstriction/vasodilation of the peripheral arteries, a heat flux sensor to measure the dissipation of heat from the body, and a two-axis accelerometer that measures motion. The data from these sensors allow Body Media to use its algorithms to calculate metabolic characteristics, activity levels, and sleep duration. The Sensewear armband has been clinically validated, and the data are organized into reports so clinicians and users can view calories burned, sleep/wake states, and activity levels among others [88]. Body Media is also developing a more detailed sleep analysis algorithm based on the data collected using the armband sensors. Using thermal characteristics and activity levels, distinctions between REM sleep and NREM sleep were made, but with a rather low sensitivity (46% for REM, 65% for NREM). However, their distinctions between sleep and wakefulness were made with a higher sensitivity (83% for wake, 93% for sleep) [89] (Figures 5.17 and 5.18).

The Sensewear armband allows convenient recording of multiple physiologic signals on a longitudinal basis, which is important in examining circadian behavior as well as metabolic characteristics. The affordable and convenient armband is non-invasive and collects multilayered datasets that provide a wealth of information without the need to visit a physician or clinical laboratory. By providing data in the natural home environment, the armband is able to give clinicians a clearer picture of physiological behavior of the individual wearing it, rather than just the snapshot of data they get during a visit to their physician [88]. However, the subject is of course required to wear the armband, introducing possible non-compliance issues

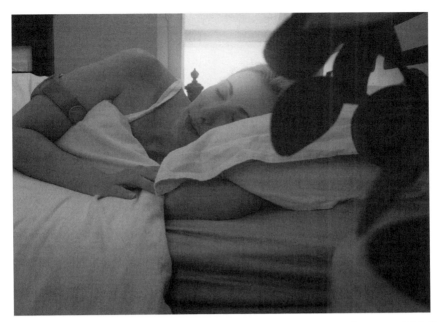

Fig. 5.17 Picture of someone wearing the armband (Image Credit: Copyright © 2007 BodyMedia, Inc. All rights reserved.)

and much of the sleep analysis performed is based on movement levels, similar to the process used by actigraphs. The algorithms that differentiate between sleep stages other than sleep/wake need to be improved before the Sensewear armband can be used to accurately assess sleep. Nonetheless, the system cannot be used to diagnose SDB.

Applications abound for this promising new device, ranging from health, wellness, and fitness to geriatrics and preventive medicine [88]. Knowing the important

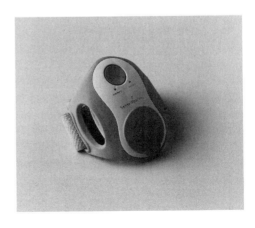

Fig. 5.18 The Sensewear® Armband (Image Credit: Copyright © 2007 BodyMedia, Inc. All rights reserved.)

physiological characteristics obtained by the armband can help physicians better target care to their patients, which leads to an improved quality of life.

5.8.7 *Tactex Fiber Optic Sensor*

Tactex Controls, Inc., in British Columbia, Canada, has developed three versions of a bed sensor including a simple occupancy-sensing device, a sensor to detect movement in bed, and another version that is able to non-invasively monitor vital signs. Their bed monitors are based on a sensitive force sensor called Kinotex® that was developed by the Canadian Space Agency for tactile robotic sensing. It is a fiber-optic-based sensor that uses two fibers (one for sending and one for receiving) embedded in a foam pad. When the foam is deformed because of a pressure change, the light is scattered differently and the return signal light intensity is changed relative to the change in pressure [90].

The design of the bed sensor allows unconstrained monitoring on many different levels to take place without disrupting the patient. It can be encased in rugged material and made durable, as Tactex has done, but the integrity of the fiber optic cables is critical to the operation of the device (90).

The first type of their bed occupancy sensors (BOS) is their basic bed alarm and occupancy sensor. This is used in hospitals and other formal care settings to alert staff when patients are entering/exiting their bed. Because the sensor goes under the mattress, there are no non-compliance issues such as patients becoming unclipped to a sensor and/or staff remembering to engage a specific sensor. The second type is the BOS-activity (ACT), an activity monitor that is able to monitor any movements that occur in bed. This is useful in determining restlessness levels of patients and gives care staff more information about the patient's quality of sleep. This is valuable especially in congregate care settings to allow the care staff to act on the information and make targeted interventions or adjustments in the patient's behavior or environment. With a non-invasive approach, the Tactex system has the potential to minimize the impact of monitoring on the patient's day-to-day activities while better informing the caregiver. The third type is the BOS-RD, designed for more comprehensive sleep research. This version is capable of detecting more subtle movements of respiration and heartbeat instead of just gross body movement or restlessness. Applications abound for this advanced technology as it is able to monitor heart rate and respiration rate based on forces from the heart's contraction and relaxation and chest wall movement, respectively. This enables the technology to be used in comprehensive sleep monitoring on a longitudinal level, or it can be used as a vital signs monitor in hospitals. Additionally, the sensor can be adapted to detect pressure points and areas that might lead to pressure sores if not relieved periodically. Providing this objective data without disturbing the patient allows nurses to be able to better monitor and treat conditions leading up to pressure sores before they become dangerous [90]. However, the diagnostic potential for this technology has not yet been proven (Figure 5.19).

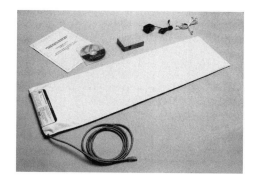

Fig. 5.19 The Tactex sensor pad (Image Credit: Copyright © 2007 Tactex Controls, Inc. All rights reserved.)

5.8.8 Air Mattress Bed Sensor

A concept based around an air mattress to record vital signs such as heart rate and respiration rate was developed at Seoul National University in South Korea by a team led by Kwangsuk Park [91]. This method is similar to one developed in Singapore by a team led by Y.T. Wang [92]. Both systems rely on a pressurized air mattress divided horizontally into different compartments. For the Korean group, the main signal for acquiring the heart rate and respiration data is derived from continuously recording the pressure differential between two of the compartments, marked by white dots as seen in Fig. 5.20. The pressure differential is generated from chest wall movements that occur during breathing and also minute forces and movements generated every time the heart contracts and relaxes. To prevent extreme pressures from developing and masking the breathing and heart rate signals during

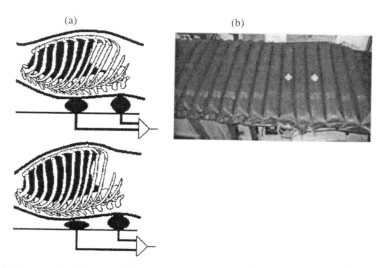

Fig. 5.20 Korean Air Mattress [91] (Image Credit: Used with permission from IOP Publishing Ltd.)

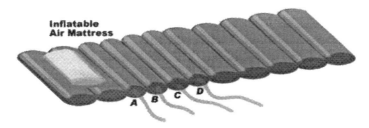

Fig. 5.21 Air Mattress from Singapore Group [92] (Image Credit: Used with permission from IOP Publishing Ltd.)

postural movement, the Korean group employed a balancing tube that has a high air resistance to equalize the pressure in the two compartments within a certain time constant. This tube also acts as a high pass filter to remove any DC signal offset after changes in position [91]. The team from Singapore takes a slightly different approach by examining the pressure differential between two compartments each for the upper chest and for the abdomen areas. As seen in Fig. 5.21, compartments A and B are used for the upper chest area whereas compartments C and D are used for the abdomen area. These differences record similar forces and movements generated from the subject lying on the mattress. Like the Korean group, the team from Singapore employs a release valve that equalizes the pressure between the two compartments for 5 s during postural movement [92].

This type of design provides an unconstrained method for monitoring different vital signs during sleep. This is important in attempting long-term sleep monitoring in natural settings without changing the routine of the subject. However, the large pressures introduced by postural movement during the night remain a drawback because they tend to mask any heartbeat or respiration signals. The balancing tube employed by the Korean group improved the performance during postural movements to an extent, but the signal quality and sensitivity remained degraded. The system also has to maintain its pressure to be functional so the system is susceptible to risk of punctures, which raises questions about the system's durability and practicality. If these issues are addressed, these two systems could be valuable in providing much needed longitudinal sleep information in a natural setting or even simply be added to a hospital bed to make it easier to get simple vital signs for a patient. Again, these diagnostic utility of these systems in assessing sleep and sleep-related disorders have not been evaluated.

5.8.9 Unconstrained Bed Sensor

A group at Hosei University in Japan led by Kajiro Watanabe has developed a pad that goes between the mattress and the frame of a bed and detects movements generated by a person sleeping on the bed. By using these movements transferred through the mattress to the pad, which is pneumatically connected to a pressure sensor, it is able to detect heartbeat, respiration, snoring, and body movements. The

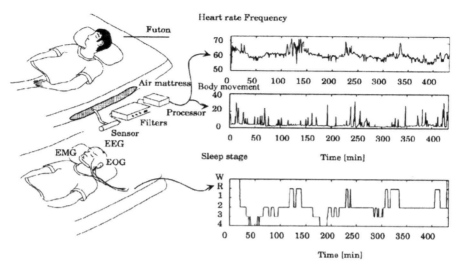

Fig. 5.22 Bed sensor developed at Hosei University [94] (Image Credit: Used with permission from IEEE and EMBS)

pad is designed to be wide enough to cover the torso area and long enough to span the width of the bed because its goal is to detect minute movements of the heart beating as well as lower frequency chest movements that are a result of breathing. The signals are processed by analog filters first and then digitally sampled at 10 Hz. A fast Fourier transform (FFT) algorithm is employed to detect the frequencies of the signals for later analysis.These FFTs are conducted using a sample of 51.2 s (for 512 points per measurement), which is then normalized to provide the data on a per minute basis. Additionally, complex statistical measures are used to take the collected data and provide basic sleep-staging information [3] (Figure 5.22).

The unconstrained design of the system provides a major advantage over any wearable technology because the user does not have to directly interact with the device. It provides a natural and non-invasive setting to collect important characteristics of sleep without requiring the user to remember to do anything outside of their normal routine. However, the sleep-staging analysis algorithms need to be further developed as initial testing did not yield good agreement [94] between this device and sleep staging conducted using the Rechschaffen and Kales method (the standard used by sleep laboratories employing EEG-based PSG). Their proposed method relies heavily on complex statistical processes and certain assumptions, which may be different when tested on people suffering from sleep disorders [94]. Moreover, the diagnostic utility of the system has not been assessed.

5.8.10 NAPS^TM

The Non-invasive Analysis of Physiological Signals (NAPS^TM) sleep analysis system, developed by the Medical Automation Research Center (MARC) at the

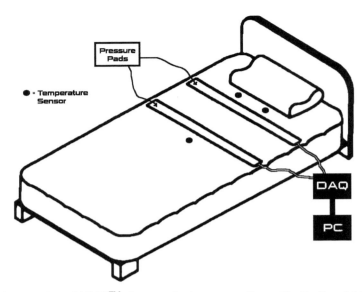

Fig. 5.23 Illustration of NAPS^{TM} sleep monitoring system (Image Credit: Copyright © 2007 Home Guardian, LLC. All rights reserved.)

University of Virginia, is a low-cost, low-power, physiological sensor-suite that can passively acquire important physiological and environmental characteristics (Figure 5.23).

It uses BCG to detect minute forces generated during cardiac contraction and relaxation, and can also detect body movement from respiratory effort and postural changes. In addition, the system can also measure environmental conditions in the immediate surroundings such as room temperature or light levels. Preliminary data [95, 96] have shown strong correlations between the heart rate passively measured using the NAPS system and conventional clinical techniques such as pulse oximetry. The NAPS system relies on a highly sensitive pressure transducer pneumatically connected to a compliant force-coupling pad installed on top of the mattress of any standard bed, on which the subject lies in order to acquire the data. Multiple pads can be used to acquire data from different parts of the body. The system is sensitive enough to gather data even when sheets and blankets are applied over the pad, which rests on the mattress. The analog signal is filtered and amplified before being digitized by A-to-D converters. An algorithm has been developed to provide automatic scoring of the instantaneous heart rate and respiration data recorded by the NAPS system. Additionally, the passive nature of the NAPS system allows data to be recorded longitudinally and to establish personalized norms for individuals that can be used to detect changes in physiological parameters, and/or to assess the efficacy of interventions [97]. Figure 5.24 shows an example comparing simultaneous EKG (top) and NAPS system waveforms. The lines between the two graphs connect the electrical impulses of the EKG to their corresponding mechanical counterparts sensed by the NAPS system.

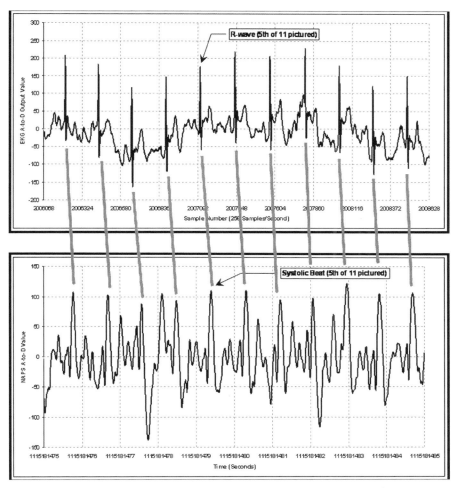

Fig. 5.24 Waveforms showing correspondence of EKG and NAPS™ System over the same 10-s period (Image Credit: Used with permission from the Medical Automation Research Center.)

The NAPS system has already proven useful as a home-health tool for qualitative sleep assessment in an assisted living environment [98]. It provided professional caregivers a better picture of their resident's sleep patterns and key information to help assess changes in their health conditions, especially when used in conjunction with other activity-monitoring equipment. Specifically, the care staff found that looking at restlessness data and sleep/wake times from the previous night's sleep helped alert them to irregularities in quality of sleep. These could indicate things such as an increase in pain or alert them to other health issues [98].

Additionally, the NAPS system is currently undergoing clinical validation against conventional PSG, the gold standard in sleep analysis. By using respiration information from two pads, one at the upper chest and one at the abdomen, the NAPS system is able to detect apneas and hypopneas along with other respiratory events. It is also able to take the entire set of physiological data and provide characteristics including heart rate and regularity, breathing rate and regularity, postural movement, and body surface temperature. These characteristics can be used to discern sleep architecture without using electrodes to monitor brain waves. In addition, other information such as sleep efficiency, TST, or additional basic sleep characteristics can be calculated from the NAPS system's data. However, the NAPS system is not able to reach the detail level of PSG (Wake, NREM, and REM sleep instead of the full six stages) because it relies on just the pneumatic pads and temperature sensors to acquire data. This limited detail level is acceptable because the NAPS system can provide this information for multiple nights, acquiring longitudinal data that will reveal sleep patterns and any changes in sleep behavior. Preliminary data analysis from a 40-subject clinical trial was conducted to make initial comparisons between the NAPS system and an EKG. Additionally, conventional PSG apnea and arousal detection were also initially compared with the NAPS system's ability to detect those events. Two 3-min segments of data were randomly selected from each subject so one segment contained no apneas or arousals and the other contained at least one event. This initial set of 4 h of data showed good agreement between the NAPS system and the conventional standards [97]. Further testing will be conducted over the entire night and a second trial will be conducted with an additional 40 subjects for the purposes of validation. Additionally, more comprehensive aspects of sleep characteristics and sleep architecture will be compared with the accepted clinical standards once the initial validation is completed.

Applications for the NAPS system are numerous as it has the versatility to be a low-cost, long-term monitoring unit for environments such as assisted living and skilled nursing facilities, while also being able to be adapted to provide a more clinical analysis of sleep over multiple nights. In the eldercare field, using the NAPS system as a monitoring tool provides objective data to nurses to target care and make adjustments in their patients' sleep behavior to increase their quality of life. It also allows them to detect health conditions early on when the NAPS system is used with daytime activity-monitoring equipment. Clinically, the NAPS system shows promise as a detailed sleep analysis tool that can provide a more non-invasive approach to sleep studies and the detection of and screening for sleep apnea. It can also be used as an outcome study tool to evaluate the effectiveness of medications and CPAP treatment along with treatment for other sleep disorders.

References

1. Summary of Findings of the 2005 Sleep in America Poll. National Sleep Foundation, 2005. (Accessed December 11, 2006, at http://www.sleepfoundation.org/_content/hottopics/2005_summary_of_findings.pdf)
2. National Sleep Disorders Research Plan. National Institutes of Health (NIH), 2003. (Accessed December 11, 2006, at http://www.nhlbi.nih.gov/health/prof/sleep/res_plan/sleep-rplan.pdf).

3. Snoring and Sleep Disorder Statistics. 2003. (Accessed December 11, 2006, at http://www.snorenet.com/education_statistics.htm).
4. Who gets obstructive sleep apnea? National Institutes of Health (NIH). (Accessed December 11, 2006, at http://www.nhlbi.nih.gov/health/dci/Diseases/SleepApnea/ SleepApnea_WhoIsAtRisk.html).
5. Kushida CA, Littner MR, Morgenthaler T, et al. Practice parameters for the indications for polysomnography and related procedures: an update for 2005. *Sleep* 2005;28(4):499–521.
6. Executive Summary of the 2003 Sleep in America Poll. National Sleep Foundation, 2003. (Accessed December 11, 2006, at http://www.sleepfoundation.org/_content/hottopics/ 2003SleepPollExecSumm.pdf).
7. ABCs of ZZZZ - When you can't sleep. National Sleep Foundation. (Accessed December 11, 2006, at http://www.sleepfoundation.org/sleeplibrary/index.php?secid=&id=53.)
8. Quan SF, et al. The Sleep Heart Health Study: design, rationale, and methods. Sleep 1997;20(12):1077–85.
9. Sleep Heart Health Study Manual of Operations. Sleep Heart Health Study Research Group. 1996. (Accessed at http://wwww.jhsph.edu/shhs)
10. Redline S, et al. Methods for obtaining and analyzing unattended polysomnography data for a multicenter study. Sleep Heart Health Research Group. Sleep 1998;21(7):759–67.
11. Nieto FJ, et al. Association of sleep-disordered breathing, sleep apnea, and hypertension in a large community-based study. Sleep Heart Health Study. *JAMA* 2000;283(14):1829–36.
12. Shahar E, et al. Sleep-disordered breathing and cardiovascular disease: cross-sectional results of the Sleep Heart Health Study. *Am J Respir Crit Care Med* 2001;163(1):19–25.
13. Mehra R, et al. Association of nocturnal arrhythmias with sleep-disordered breathing: The Sleep Heart Health Study. *Am J Respir Crit Care Med* 2006;173(8):910–6.
14. Punjabi NM, et al. Sleep-disordered breathing, glucose intolerance, and insulin resistance: the Sleep Heart Health Study. *Am J Epidemiol* 2004;160(6):521–30.
15. Gottlieb DJ, et al. Does snoring predict sleepiness independently of apnea and hypopnea frequency? *Am J Respir Crit Care Med* 2000;162(4 Pt 1):1512–7.
16. Baldwin CM, et al. The association of sleep-disordered breathing and sleep symptoms with quality of life in the Sleep Heart Health Study. *Sleep* 2001;24(1):96–105.
17. Young T, et al. Predictors of sleep-disordered breathing in community-dwelling adults: the Sleep Heart Health Study. *Arch Intern Med* 2002;162(8):893–900.
18. Walsleben JA, et al. Sleep and reported daytime sleepiness in normal subjects: the Sleep Heart Health Study. *Sleep* 2004;27(2):293–8.
19. Aserinsky E, Kleitman N. Regularly occurring periods of eye motility, and concomitant phenomena, during sleep. *Science* 1953;118(3062):273–4.
20. Dement W, Kleitman N. Cyclic variations in EEG during sleep and their relation to eye movements, body motility, and dreaming. *Electroencephalogr Clin Neurophysiol Suppl* 1957;9(4):673–90.
21. Gastaut H, Tassinari CA, Duron B. [Polygraphic study of diurnal and nocturnal (hypnic and respiratory) episodal manifestations of Pickwick syndrome]. *Rev Neurol (Paris)* 1965;112(6):568–79.
22. Jung R, Kuhlo W. Neurophysiological studies of abnormal night sleep and the Pickwickian syndrome. *Prog Brain Res* 1965;18:140–59.
23. Dement W. History of sleep physiology and medicine. In: Kryger M, Roth, T., Dement, W., eds. *Principles and Practice of Sleep Medicine*, 4th ed. Philadelphia: Saunders; 2005:1–12.
24. Rechtschaffen A, Kales, A. (eds.). A manual of standardized terminology: techniques and scoring system for sleep stages of human subjects. Los Angeles: UCLA Brain Information/Brain Research Institute; 1968.
25. Kapur VK, et al. Rates of sensor loss in unattended home polysomnography: the influence of age, gender, obesity, and sleep-disordered breathing. *Sleep* 2000;23(5):682–8.
26. Whitney CW, et al. Reliability of scoring respiratory disturbance indices and sleep staging. *Sleep* 1998;21(7):749–57.

27. Centers for Medicare & Medicaid Services. (Accessed January 29, 2007, at www.cms.hhs.gov).
28. Hirshkowitz M, Kryger, M. Monitoring techniques for evaluating suspected sleep-disordered breathing. In: Kryger M, Roth, T, Dement, W, eds. *Principles and Practice of Sleep Medicine*, 4th ed. Philadelphia: Saunders; 2005:1378–1393.
29. Sleep-related breathing disorders in adults: recommendations for syndrome definition and measurement techniques in clinical research. The Report of an American Academy of Sleep Medicine Task Force. Sleep 1999;22(5):667–89.
30. Carskadon MA, et al. Guidelines for the multiple sleep latency test (MSLT): a standard measure of sleepiness. *Sleep* 1986;9(4):519–24.
31. Haponik EF, et al. Evaluation of sleep-disordered breathing. Is polysomnography necessary? *Am J Med* 1984;77(4):671–7.
32. Arias A, et al. Diagnostic yield of daytime nap polysomnography. *Am Rev Respir Dis* 1992;145:A724.
33. Chesson AL, Jr., et al. The indications for polysomnography and related procedures. *Sleep* 1997;20(6):423–87.
34. Ferber R, et al. Portable recording in the assessment of obstructive sleep apnea. ASDA standards of practice. *Sleep* 1994;17(4):378–92.
35. Portier F, et al. Evaluation of home versus laboratory polysomnography in the diagnosis of sleep apnea syndrome. *Am J Respir Crit Care Med* 2000;162(3 Pt 1):814–8.
36. Fry JM, et al. Full polysomnography in the home. *Sleep* 1998;21(6):635–42.
37. Flemons WW, et al. Home diagnosis of sleep apnea: a systematic review of the literature. An evidence review cosponsored by the American Academy of Sleep Medicine, the American College of Chest Physicians, and the American Thoracic Society. *Chest* 2003;124(4):1543–79.
38. Iber C, et al. Single night studies in obstructive sleep apnea. *Sleep* 1991;14(5):383–5.
39. Sadeh A, et al. The role of actigraphy in the evaluation of sleep disorders. *Sleep* 1995;18(4):288–302.
40. Tryon WW. *Activity Measurement in Psychology and Medicine*. New York: Plenum Press; 1991.
41. Kupfer DJ, et al. Psychomotor activity in affective states. *Arch Gen Psychiatry* 1974;30(6):765–8.
42. McPartland R, Kupfer, D, Foster, F. The movement-activated recording monitor: third generation motor-activity monitoring system. *Behav Res Methods Instrum* 1976;8:357–60.
43. Colburn TR, et al. An ambulatory activity monitor with solid state memory. *ISA Trans* 1976;15(2):149–54.
44. Ancoli-Israel S. Actigraphy. In: Kryger M, Roth, T, Dement, W, eds. *Principles and Practice of Sleep Medicine*, 3rd ed. Philadelphia: W. B. Saunders Company; 2000:1295–301.
45. Redmond D, Hegge, FW. Observations on the design and specification of a wrist-worn human activity monitoring system. *Behav Res Methods Instr Comput* 1985;17:659–69.
46. Borbély AA. Long-term recording of the rest-activity cycle in man. In: Zbinden G, Cuomo, V, Racagni, G, et al., eds. *Application of Behavioral Pharmacology in Toxicology*. New York: Raven Press; 1983:39–44.
47. Borbély AA. New techniques for the analysis of the human sleep-wake cycle. *Brain Dev* 1986;8:482–8.
48. Ancoli-Israel S, et al. The role of actigraphy in the study of sleep and circadian rhythms. *Sleep* 2003;26(3):342–92.
49. Starr I, Noordergraaf A. *Ballistocardiography in Cardiovascular Research; Physical Aspects of the Circulation in Health and Disease*. Amsterdam: North-Holland Pub. Co.; 1967.
50. Stead EA, Jr. An appreciation of Isaac Starr. *N Engl J Med* 1979;300(16):930–1.
51. Polo O. Partial upper airway obstruction during sleep. Studies with the static charge-sensitive bed (SCSB). *Acta Physiol Scand Suppl* 1992;606:1–118.
52. Harrison WK, Talbot SA. Two new forms of ultra-low frequency ballistocardiograph. *Bibl Cardiol* 1967(19):13–8.

53. Nyboer J, Reid KA, Gessert W. A servo counterforce ballistocardiograph. An aperiodic air-bearing system. *Bibl Cardiol* 1967(19):26–32.
54. Tolles WE. Computer search for ballistocardiographic indices of cardiovascular disease. *Bibl Cardiol* 1967(19):126–35.
55. Scarborough WR, Podolak E, Whitlock MB. Magnetic tape recording of ballistocardiograms and other physiologic variables from subjects with and without cardiovascular "disease". *Bibl Cardiol* 1967(19):72–98.
56. Trefny Z, Wagner J. A quantitative ballistocardiograph. *Bibl Cardiol* 1967(19):19–25.
57. Goedhard WJ. Ballistocardiography: past, present and future. *Bibl Cardiol* 1979(37):27–45.
58. Iber C, et al. Polysomnography performed in the unattended home versus the attended laboratory setting–Sleep Heart Health Study methodology. *Sleep* 2004;27(3):536–40.
59. Quan SF, et al. Short-term variablility of respiration and sleep during unattended nonlaboratory polysomnogaphy–the Sleep Heart Health Study. *Sleep* 2002;25(8):843–9.
60. Su S, et al. A comparison of polysomnography and a portable home sleep study in the diagnosis of obstructive sleep apnea syndrome. *Otolaryngol Head Neck Surg* 2004;131:844–50.
61. Collop NA. Portable monitoring for diagnosing obstructive sleep apnea: not yet ready for primetime. *Chest* 2004;125(3):809–11.
62. Liesching TN, et al. Evaluation of the accuracy of SNAP technology sleep sonography in detecting obstructive sleep apnea in adults compared to standard polysomnography. *Chest* 2004;125(3):886–91.
63. Verse T, et al. Validation of the POLY-MESAM seven-channel ambulatory recording unit. *Chest* 2000;117(6):1613–8.
64. Epstein LJ, Dorlac GR. Cost-effectiveness analysis of nocturnal oximetry as a method of screening for sleep apnea-hypopnea syndrome. *Chest* 1998;113(1):97–103.
65. Hussain SF, Fleetham JA. Overnight home oximetry: Can it identify patients with obstructive sleep apnea-hypopnea who have minimal daytime sleepiness? *Respir Med* 2003;97(5):537–40.
66. Chiner E, et al. Nocturnal oximetry for the diagnosis of the sleep apnoea hypopnoea syndrome: A method to reduce the number of polysomnographies? *Thorax* 1999;54(11):968–71.
67. Issa FG, et al. Digital monitoring of sleep-disordered breathing using snoring sound and arterial oxygen saturation. *Am Rev Respir Dis* 1993;148(4 Pt 1):1023–9.
68. AMI: Physiological Actigraph monitoring of ambulatory subjects for sleep, psychiatric and movement disorders via Actigraphy. Ambulatory Monitoring, Inc. (Accessed December 11, 2006, at www.ambulatory-monitoring.com)
69. Mini Mitter: Actigraphs and Biotelemetric Physiological Monitors for Humans and Animals. Mini Mitter. (Accessed December 11, 2006, at www.minimitter.com)
70. Benson K, et al. The measurement of sleep by actigraphy: direct comparison of 2 commercially available actigraphs in a nonclinical population. *Sleep* 2004;27(5):986–9.
71. Alihanka J, Vaahtoranta K. A static charge sensitive bed. A new method for recording body movements during sleep. *Electroencephalogr Clin Neurophysiol* 1979;46(6):731–4.
72. Alihanka J, Vaahtoranta K, Saarikivi I. A new method for long-term monitoring of the ballistocardiogram, heart rate, and respiration. *Am J Physiol* 1981;240(5):R384–92.
73. Erkinjuntti M, et al. Use of the SCSB method for monitoring of respiration, body movements and ballistocardiogram in infants. *Early Hum Dev* 1984;9(2):119–26.
74. Jansen BH, Shankar K. Sleep staging with movement-related signals. *Int J Biomed Comput* 1993;32(3–4):289–97.
75. Penzel T, et al. MESAM: a heart rate and snoring recorder for detection of obstructive sleep apnea. *Sleep* 1990;13(2):175–82.
76. Penzel T, et al. A device for ambulatory heart rate, oxygen saturation and snoring recording. In: *Annual International Conference of the IEEE Engineering in Medicine and Biology Society (EMBS)*; 1991; pp. 1616–7.
77. Esnaola S, et al. Diagnostic accuracy of a portable recording device (MESAM IV) in suspected obstructive sleep apnoea. *Eur Respir J* 1996;9(12):2597–605.
78. van der Loos HFM, et al. Unobtrusive Vital Signs Monitoring from a Multisensor Bed Sheet. In: *RESNA 2001*, Reno, NV; June 22–26, 2001, p. 218–220.

79. SleepSmart. Spark Works Engineering. (Accessed 2003, at www.spark-works.com)

80. van der Loos HFM, Ullrich, N, Kobayashi, H. Development of sensate and robotic bed technologies for vital signs monitoring and sleep quality improvement. *Autonomous Robots* 2003;15:67–79.

81. Watch PAT 100. Itamar Medical Ltd. (Accessed December 11, 2006, at http://www.itamar-medical.com/objects/WatchPat100F.pdf).

82. Itamar Medical Information: Watch PAT 100. Itamar Medical Ltd. (Accessed December 11, 2006, at http://www.itamar-medical.com/content.asp?id=31).

83. Ayas NT, et al. Assessment of a wrist-worn device in the detection of obstructive sleep apnea. *Sleep Med* 2003;4(5):435–42.

84. Herscovici S, et al. Picking REM from the Finger–Further Improvement of the Algorithm Using an Advanced Predicting Function. In: *SLEEP 2006*; Salt Lake City, UT; 2006;29: p. A343.

85. Apnea Risk Evaluation System (ARES). Advanced Brain Monitoring, Inc. (Accessed December 11, 2006, at http://www.b-alert.com/ARES.html).

86. Westbrook PR, et al. Description and validation of the apnea risk evaluation system: a novel method to diagnose sleep apnea-hypopnea in the home. *Chest* 2005;128(4):2166–75.

87. Ayappa I, et al. Validation of a Self-applied Unattended Monitor for Sleep Disordered Breathing (SDB). In: *SLEEP* 2006; Salt Lake City, UT; 2006; 29: p. A343–44.

88. BodyMedia Body Monitoring System. BodyMedia, Inc. (Accessed December 11, 2006, at http://www.bodymedia.com/pdf/brochure_bms.pdf).

89. Germain A, Buysse, DJ, Kupfer, DJ. Preliminary Validation of New Device for Studying Sleep. In: *SLEEP 2006*; Salt Lake City, UT; 2006. p. A351.

90. Tactile Force Sensors. Tactex Controls, Inc. (Accessed December 11, 2006, at www.tactex.com).

91. Chee Y, Han J, Youn J, Park K. Air mattress sensor system with balancing tube for unconstrained measurement of respiration and heart beat movements. *Physiol Meas* 2005;26(4):413–22.

92. Chow P, et al. Respiratory monitoring using an air-mattress system. *Physiol Meas* 2000;21(3):345–54.

93. Watanabe K, et al. Noninvasive measurement of heartbeat, respiration, snoring and body movements of a subject in bed via a pneumatic method. *IEEE Trans Biomed Eng* 2005;52(12):2100–7.

94. Watanabe T, Watanabe K. Noncontact method for sleep stage estimation. *IEEE Trans Biomed Eng* 2004;51(10):1735–48.

95. Mack DC, et al. Non-invasive analysis of physiological signals (NAPS): a low cost passive monitor for sleep quality and related applications. In: *Carillion Biomedical Institute Steps to Success Conference*; 2002 October; Roanoke, VA: Carillion Biomedical Institute; 2002.

96. Mack DC, et al. Non-invasive analysis of physiological signals (NAPS): a vibration sensor that passively detects heart and respiration as a part of a sensor suite for medical monitoring. In: *Summer Bioengineering Conference*; 2003 June 25–29; Key Biscayne, FL; 2003.

97. Mack DC, et al. A passive and portable system for monitoring heart rate and detecting sleep apnea and arousals: preliminary validation. In: *Distributed Diagnosis and Home Healthcare (D2H2)*; Conference 2006 April 2–4; Arlington, VA: IEEE; 2006.

98. Alwan M, et al. Impact of monitoring technology in assisted living: outcome pilot. *IEEE Trans Inf Technol Biomed* 2006;10(1):192–8.

Chapter 6
Vision Impairment Assessment and Assistive Technologies

Stanley Woo

6.1 Background

Low vision refers to a condition of irreversible vision loss that is not correctable by conventional spectacles, contact lenses, surgery, or medicine. The ocular disease leads to a visual impairment that results in a functional limitation of the eye or visual system. This may include a reduction in detail vision (visual acuity), side vision (peripheral visual field), distorted or double vision, or a combination thereof. The consequence of this impairment may lead to a visual disability that prevents the person from performing specific tasks such as reading, driving, cooking, or watching television. Depending on the severity of the disability, the result may be a visual handicap that may lead to a loss of personal and/or socioeconomic independence. Much work has been done in an attempt to classify the interaction of visual impairment, disability, and handicap in an effort to characterize the impact of low-vision rehabilitation (LVR) as a treatment modality [1, 2]. LVR embraces an inter-disciplinary approach to ameliorating the handicap and maximizing quality of life for the partially sighted [3].

Eligibility for services for the elderly for LVR often depends on categorizing the level of visual impairment, specifically whether a person is "legally blind" or "visually impaired." The Social Security Administration defines "legal blindness" as best corrected visual acuity in the better seeing eye that is 20/200 or worse. Alternatively, it may be characterized by a visual field less than 20° in diameter in the eye with the larger remaining field [4]. Visual impairment describes vision that does not meet the criteria for legal blindness but may still result in a visual disability or handicap. These are codified in the "International Classification of Diseases, 9th Revision, Clinical Modification" (ICD-9-CM), Sixth Edition, based on the combination of vision (visual acuity and/or visual field) in each eye. The ICD-9 codes are essential for documentation and billing for rehabilitative services (Table 6.1).

Stanley Woo
Clinical Associate Professor, Chief, Low Vision Rehabilitation Services, Director, Center for Sight Enhancement, University of Houston College of Optometry, Houston, TX 77204-2020
e-mail: SWoo@OPTOMETRY.UH.EDU

From: *Aging Medicine, Eldercare Technology for Clinical Practitioners,*
Edited by: M. Alwan and R. Felder © Humana Press, Totowa, NJ

Table 6.1 ICD-9 codes for visual impairment and legal blindness

		Impairment level of better eye						
		Total impairment	Near-Total impairment	Profound impairment	Severe impairment	Moderate impairment	Near-normal visual acuity	Normal visual acuity
		NLP	<20/1000	20/500–20/1000	20/200–20/400	20/70–20/160	20/30–20/60	20/10–20/25
			≤5°	≤10°	≤20°			
Impairment level of lesser eye	Total impairment NLP	369.01	369.03	369.06	369.12	369.16	369.62	369.63
	Near-total impairment <20/1000 ≤5°		369.04	369.07	369.13	369.17	369.65	369.66
	Profound impairment 20/500–20/1000 ≤10°			369.08	369.14	369.18	369.68	369.69
	Severe impairment 20/200–20/400 ≤20°				369.22	369.24	369.72	369.73
	Moderate impairment 20/70–20/160					369.25	369.75	369.76

Regrettably, the label "legal blindness" is a misnomer that does a disservice to the visually impaired population, because it emphasizes the vision loss rather than the potential to be realized from the significant, remaining functional vision. Furthermore, it reinforces the stigma and myth that nothing more can be done to help their vision. The LVR team may consist of an optometrist in a role analogous to the physiatrist in physical medicine, along with an ophthalmologist, occupational therapist, certified low-vision therapist, social worker, and psychologist, among others. By integrating the diagnosis, treatment, and rehabilitation of the individual, appropriate prescriptive decisions can be made regarding optical, electronic, and non-optical adaptive aids that may assist the partially sighted to optimize the use of remaining vision to treat the visual disability and handicap. A challenge for providers of elder care in optometry is to raise awareness that LVR may provide a treatment option in the standard of care.

6.2 Demographics, Eye Disease, and Prevalence of Low Vision

Estimates of the number of visually impaired in the USA range from roughly 3.3 million to 13.5 million people [5, 6]. The leading causes of vision loss in North America include age-related macular degeneration (AMD), diabetic retinopathy, glaucoma, and cataracts. AMD is a retinal disease that has a predilection for the photoreceptors responsible for central detail vision. It results in decreased visual acuity but spares peripheral vision. Diabetic retinopathy is a retinal disease that affects the small blood vessels of the retina and may result in loss of visual acuity and peripheral vision and if left untreated, may lead to blindness. Glaucoma is a disease that affects the optic nerve, which may result in a gradual decrease in peripheral vision and visual acuity. Cataracts are a yellowing and hardening of the crystalline lens over time and may impact contrast sensitivity; however, this condition may be treated with surgery. Using an intraocular lens implant, some with accommodative properties, may restore vision if the retina remains healthy.

Age-related eye diseases resulting in irreversible vision loss are chronic and progressive and vary by ethnicity. According to results from the Eye Disease Prevalence Research Group, the leading cause of blindness in Caucasians is AMD with an estimated prevalence of 56.4%. In Blacks, the leading causes were cataracts (36.8%) and glaucoma (26.0%). Lastly, in Hispanics the leading cause was glaucoma (28.6%) [5]. Irrespective of ethnicity, the prevalence of visual impairment increases with age from about 0.31% in those between 40 and 50 years of age to over 23% in those over 80 years of age [5]. With longer life expectancies, the National Center for Health Statistics estimates that the number of visually impaired will double within the next decade. Sadly, it is estimated that less than 25% of the visually impaired have received comprehensive LVR services [3].

6.3 Identifying Patient Goals and Visual Objectives

Along with the standard case history including review of systems, the LVR eval-uation emphasizes the patient's visual goals and objectives. Specificity in visual task identification is important because different adaptive aids and techniques may be necessary to accomplish their goals. In the past, the patient may have simply updated their spectacle prescription to address all their visual needs. Assessing a patient's affect and motivation is also important to establish early in the evaluation as the prognosis for a successful outcome is dependent on both. For instance, we may have one patient who presents with AMD and a visual acuity of 20/70 but reports that he or she is "completely blind" and has given up reading and cooking. Counseling to emphasize the significant amount of vision remaining is critical. In addition, the patient may be reassured by the fact that using their vision will not accelerate or exacerbate the disease process. In other words, there is no advantage to avoiding visual tasks to conserve their vision. At the other end of the spectrum, we may have another patient with AMD who presents with visual acuity of 20/400 and reports that they simply need the "eye specialist report" signed to renew their driver's license. Counseling about their current expectations and the relationship to external agencies such as the Department of Public Safety/Department of Motor Vehicles may be important. Fortunately, the majority present with expectations somewhere in between, and the case history is an excellent opportunity to educate the patient about the rehabilitative process along with expectations and outcomes.

A functional visual history may explore tasks such as reading in more detail to elucidate key goals. For instance, short-term spot reading of mail, bills, and med-ications is a very different task than reading journal articles, paperback novels, or newspaper. Other tasks that may not be traditionally addressed include personal hygiene, grooming, cooking, seeing stove dials, and thermostats, among others. Massof et al. explore a systematic approach to goal and task identification using a hierarchical system and Rasch analysis [2, 7]. Ultimately, the list of tasks can be overwhelming and time consuming, thus necessitating the use of survey instruments to improve efficiency without losing essential information. One of the most widely used instruments in LVR is the Vision Function Questionnaire-25 (NEI-VFQ-25) developed by the National Eye Institute [8]. The NEI-VFQ-25 is a survey of self-reported vision-targeted health status that includes task-oriented domains, along with emotional well-being and social functioning questions. Scoring results in an initial index of global visual function along with sub-scales for distance and near activities that can serve as a baseline functional measure.

The case history is an excellent opportunity to establish rapport with the patient and counsel them on the rehabilitative process. Too often, patients are seeking a quick fix with "magic glasses" that they believe will restore their vision. By empha-sizing the amount of functional vision remaining and counseling them about the adaptive aids and techniques necessary to achieve their goals, they may begin the work necessary for them to master their objectives. The case history also provides an opportunity to be proactive in addressing potentially sensitive areas such as Charles Bonnet syndrome (CBS). CBS is characterized by non-threatening visual hallucinations associated with visual impairment [9, 10]. Patients are aware that the things that they see are not real, such as flowers in the middle of the driveway, teapots on the television, and the like. CBS has likely been under-reported because of concern that this may be related to early dementia or Alzheimer's. However, no such association has been established, and the resulting relief for the patient and their caregivers is often substantial.

6.4 Clinical Visual Assessment

Visual function varies with age, and several measures beyond simple visual acuity are necessary to characterize visual function [11]. In particular, visual acuity, contrast sensitivity, and visual field testing yield useful clinical information that impacts LVR.

6.4.1 Visual Acuity

Visual acuity is the standard vision performance measure that quantifies central detail vision. It is an angular measure of the resolving ability of the neuro-optical system [12]. Distance visual acuity may be measured by a number of different charts including the Snellen projector, Bailey-Lovie, Early Treatment of Diabetic Retinopathy Study (ETDRS), and Feinbloom number chart. Computer display charts such as the B-VAT (Medtronic, ENT, Jacksonville, FL) are becoming increasingly common place with the advantages of being able to manipulate contrast and provide a wide range of optotypes with different presentation formats. Visual acuity is often represented as a ratio of test distance over letter size. For example, a patient with "normal vision" may be able to see 20/20; however, a patient with AMD may see 20/200. The significance of this ratio is that the patient with AMD in this case must stand at 20 feet to see what the "reference" observer can see at 200 feet. As many low-vision patients are often unable to see even the big "E" on a standard projector chart, hand-held charts with more intervals in letter size are often used at a distance of 10 feet to provide a more accurate measurement.

Near visual acuity and reading are similarly assessed at the patient's habitual distance and serve as a basis for estimation of magnification required to see the target size text. Single letters with high contrast represent the optimal near visual acuity (NVA), whereas continuous text charts may better represent reading performance. There are a number of cards available including the Lighthouse single letter chart, Feinbloom paragraph card, and the MNRead card. Reduced Snellen scoring for near acuity loses its meaning when tested at distances other than 40 cm and should thus be avoided. In other words, a 20/50 acuity at near typically applies to a reference distance of 40 cm. However, if the patient were to hold the card closer at 20 cm to read the 20/50 line, the actual acuity equivalent would be 20/100. The ambiguity of this metric is alleviated by adoption of the M system for near visual acuity developed by Sloan [13]. The M system is standardized such that the "x-height" of a lower case letter subtends 5 min of arc at a distance of 1 m. Thus, a 1M letter is 1.45 mm tall, which approximates newspaper size print. By measuring the test distance, a more accurate measurement of near VA facilitates the process of magnification estimation. In estimating magnification, variations in target size print vary with the task (Table 6.2). For the older population, it is imperative that these measurements be made with the bifocal portion of the glasses or single vision readers to provide optimal focus.

6.4.2 Reading Performance

Reading is a complex task that includes factors such as acuity reserve, contrast reserve, and field of view [15, 16]. The importance of these parameters is to recognize that calculations of magnification typically begin at threshold but should factor in a reserve to facilitate optimal performance. If an older adult with 20/20 vision were to attempt to read the fine print on a lease or contract (0.5M), they would likely be able to do so. However, as it is very close to their threshold, the reading would be slow and labored. Consequently, providing additional magnification to read print smaller than the target size has the benefit of improving reading performance.

The MNRead acuity chart is a reading performance test, which can measure both visual acuity and reading speed. Arranged in a log scale, the card may be held at various distances with predictable changes in measured acuity [17]. Furthermore, maximum reading speed may be estimated from super-threshold targets, and as the print size gets smaller, reading speed drops off. This inflection point is referred to as the critical print size and represents the smallest print size at which the patient can read at their maximum rate [18]. The result is representative of the target performance level to be expected upon successful LVR.

A practical observation noted in patients with asymmetrical acuity is the tendency to close one eye while reading. Although one would assume that the eye with better vision would simply dominate the binocular percept, it has been observed that binocular rivalry may contribute to symptoms such as losing one's place and having

Table 6.2 Common print sizes [14]

M size	Red Snellen at 40 cm	Point size	Common text size
10 M	20/500	80	1/2" letters
5 M	20/250	40	Newspaper headlines
4 M	20/200	32	Newspaper subheadline
2 M	20/100	16	Children's books, large print
1.6 M	20/80	12	Children's books
1.2 M	20/60	10	Magazine print
1 M	20/50	8	Text Books, newspaper print
0.8 M	20/40	6	Paperback, newspaper print
0.6 M	20/32	5	Newspaper print, stocks
0.5 M	20/25	4	Small bible, footnotes
0.4 M	20/20	3	

the words run together. Occluding the worse eye during reading often improves reading performance with the appropriate adaptive device. With training and experience, patients may be able to wean themselves off of the monocular occlusion.

6.4.3 Contrast Sensitivity and Glare

The limitation of visual acuity as a measure of visual performance is that it measures a single point at high contrast. However, the real world requires functional vision that reflects a percept that varies in both contrast and spatial frequency. Contrast is defined as $(L_{max} - L_{min})/(L_{max} + L_{min})$, where L_{max} and L_{min} are the luminance maximum and minimum, respectively. LVR often includes tests of contrast sensitivity function (CSF), particularly when symptoms such as missing steps, curbs, and other similar mobility concerns arise.

There are a number of clinical tests for contrast sensitivity including the Bailey-Lovie high–low contrast chart, the Pelli-Robson chart, and Mars chart. Each has a number of strengths and ultimately correlates with various domains within the contrast-sensitivity function. The clinical utility of the results are predictive of mobility concerns and also subsequent reading performance [19].

Another important consideration in the elderly eye is that "the 60-year-old retina receives approximately one-third of the amount of light which reaches the 20-year-old retina" [20]. Thus, elderly people with no visual impairment require significantly higher light levels than young normal subjects to optimize performance. However, there are cases where decreased illumination must be considered because of photophobia and/or glare.

Glare or dazzling is a sense of excessive brightness within the visual field that can impair visual performance (disability glare) or may simply create discomfort (discomfort glare). Disability glare depends on the luminance of the glare source relative to that of the object of regard and on the angular separation (ϕ) between them. The effect of a peripheral glare source on the retinal image is to decrease contrast by raising the overall illumination level while maintaining the absolute luminance difference between adjacent regions of the image. Selective wavelength cut-off filters may result in significant subjective relief of asthenopic symptoms associated with both poor contrast sensitivity and glare.

6.4.4 Visual Fields

Visual field testing can quantify both the extent and the sensitivity of remaining visual function. Automated testing uses sophisticated algorithms to plot out the hill of vision to assist in the rehabilitation plan. Various strategies may be used depending on the area of interest and type of disease under study including AMD, glaucoma, and stroke. More recently, scanning laser technology has been applied so that specific spots on the retina may be evaluated in real time to provide more immediate feedback during evaluation and training. These tests of visual field are in-office procedures.

To monitor changes in central field loss at home, an Amsler grid is commonly used. The paper test consists of a target grid that subtends the central 20° when held at a distance of 30 cm. By directing their attention to the center of the grid, the patient may notice areas or lines that are wavy and/or missing. These correspond to areas affected by AMD. By testing one eye at a time, one is able to monitor changes on a daily basis and to seek care sooner than scheduled as needed. Various studies have indicated that the sensitivity of the test is limited, but no superior alternative has yet been developed.

6.4.5 Low-Vision Refraction

Patients with ocular disease may often come in with glasses that are several years old or report that their previous eye care provider has been reluctant to make any updates in the spectacle prescription. Consequently, in pursuit of treatment of the disease alone, the refractive status of a patient may end up neglected at worst or a diminished priority at best. For those patients with substantial opacities or difficulty with eccentric viewing (EV), trial frame refraction may provide substantial improvement in visual performance as a result of having an accurate spectacle prescription. Tools that are readily available to estimate the initial magnitude, such as retinoscopy or auto-refraction, are a good starting point. However, in cases where dense opacities or patient compliance are difficult, the astute clinician may turn to trial frame refraction.

The refraction is facilitated by technology such as auto-refractors and refined by applying the principle of the just-noticeable difference (JND). "The JND is that amount of spherical lens change at which a change in clarity or blur is first noticed" [21]. The JND serves as a convenient rule of thumb for estimating the necessary dioptric power change. Some of the advantages of the trial frame versus a traditional refraction behind the phoropter include the adoption of more natural compensatory postures and strategies. For instance, in the presence of central field loss in AMD, a patient may wish to adopt an EV position. This facilitates measurement of more accurate VA and reinforces the patient's perception about whether a change in spectacles may truly be of benefit. An accurate spectacle prescription is the platform upon which functional vision may be maximized.

6.5 Low-Vision Rehabilitation

6.5.1 Principles of Magnification

In the presence of central visual field loss, a decrease in visual acuity is anticipated. As the size of the lesion increases, greater detail vision is lost. EV is used to direct remaining functional vision onto the target of regard; however, to be resolved, the print must be magnified. Magnification may be accomplished by a number of strategies including relative distance, relative size, angular, and electronic [22, 23].

Relative distance simply involves moving the target closer to the eye resulting in an increased retinal image size. Concurrent focusing for the closer distance is necessary to optimize clarity along with the increased retinal image size. Relative size magnification involves making the target text larger as in Reader's Digest Large Print or photocopying text at 200%. Angular magnification uses lenses and optical characteristics to create a larger angular subtense of the image at the eye relative to the original object. Telescopes are an example of the use of angular magnification. Lastly, electronic magnification may be achieved by using a closed circuit camera and projecting an electronic image of the target text to a display [cathode ray tube (CRT) or LCD]. The resulting image may be magnified and the contrast manipulated and enhanced to provide improved readability.

Identifying the appropriate adaptive aid should be based on an interpretation of the clinical data including pathology, visual objective, and physical characteristics of the patient to maximize efficiency and the probability for a successful outcome. Initial reaction to magnification may be determined from loose lenses following trial frame refraction. By identifying the appropriate corrective power to read the target size print, the question of what magnifier to choose follows a rational determination rather than a random affair. Furthermore, early success encourages the patient to recognize the visual potential to accomplish the goal.

Conventional magnification is measured in terms of "x" and is a comparison of the size of the image viewed by the magnifier relative to the object at a reference distance of 25 cm. The reciprocal of this reference distance can be stated in terms of lens or dioptric power (D), where the reciprocal of 25 cm corresponds to +4D. The power of the magnifier divided by four thus relates to the magnification in terms of "x." For example, a +24D lens would be more commonly known as a 6× magnifier. The actual application of the formula becomes more complex with different platforms for adaptive aids. For instance, a 6× stand magnifier as labeled by the manufacturer will provide a variable amount of magnification as the patient's eye to lens distance varies. The detail of the optics of these devices is beyond the scope of this chapter; however, it should be realized that magnification estimation should have a solid theoretical foundation to assure the greatest probability for a successful outcome.

6.5.2 Optical Devices for Near Visual Objectives

Once the appropriate amount of magnification has been determined, a number of adaptive devices may be evaluated to determine their efficacy in achieving the desired outcome. High-power spectacle lenses, also known as microscopes, may be able to assist with prolonged reading tasks using a portable and relatively lightweight system. Advances in optical design have improved field of view while

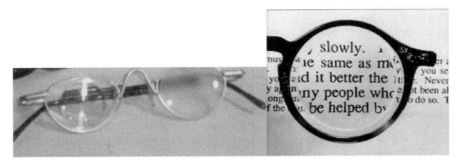

Fig. 6.1 (Left) Microsope with diffractive optics (Noves, Eschenbach) for reading. (Right) Microscope using doublet optics (ClearImage II, Designs for Vision, Inc.)

decreasing weight, thickness, and aberrations and include diffractive optics and doublet designs (Figure 6.1).

In higher powers over +8D, it is often advisable to correct for the better seeing eye rather than to attempt to achieve binocularity. The principal advantage of microscopes is the relatively large field of view. The principal disadvantage is that the microscope often focuses at a relatively close distance to read, which may prove troublesome for some elderly people (Table 6.3). This may be overcome in part by having the patient begin at their nose with the material and push out gradually until the print becomes clear. With additional training and good lighting, spectacle microscopes provide an excellent option for prolonged reading tasks.

For short-term spot reading, hand-held illuminated magnifiers provide a wide range of options (Figure 6.2). Lighting options include incandescent and halogen bulbs along with newer light-emitting diodes (LED). As the power of the magnifier increases, the diameter of the lens typically decreases resulting in a smaller field of view. There are a number of manufacturers and distributors of hand-held magnifiers including Eschenbach, Optelec (Chelmsford, MA), Lighthouse, Schweizer, among others. The challenge for the optometrist is finding the optimal balance between magnification and field of view in light of the patients' vision and objectives. These

Table 6.3 Approximate focal lengths of common lens powers

Power (D)	Distance		Power (D)	Distance	
	cm	inches		Cm	inches
+1.00	100		+8.00	13	
+1.50	67		+10.00	10	4"
+2.00	50		+12.00	8	
+2.50	40	16"	+14.00	7	
+2.75	36		+16.00	6	
+3.00	33		+20.00	5	2"
+3.50	29		+24.00	4	
+4.00	25		+28.00	3.5	
+5.00	20	8"	+32.00	3	
+6.00	17		+40.00	2.5	1"

Fig. 6.2 Hand-held illuminated magnifier demonstrating enlarged image of the scale on a syringe used for insulin injection

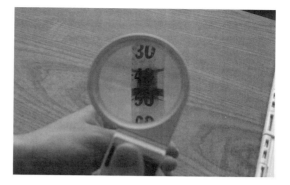

devices are ideal for reading medicine labels, stove dials, microwave display panels, mail, and bills. In addition, their portability and light source provide enhanced capability to read price labels and menus.

Stand magnifiers provide a relatively stable platform as the lens rest on top of the reading material (Figure 6.3). Again, a number of lighting options are available including incandescent, halogen, xenon, and LED. This may be accomplished by using handles equipped with either batteries or a plug-in transformer. As the power of a stand magnifier increases, the width of the lens decreases to minimize weight and thickness. This results in a smaller field of view, which can be overcome in part by holding the magnifier closer to the eye. The magnifier itself enlarges the target by creating a virtual, erect image, which necessitates the use of a bifocal segment for optimal focus. One problem that may arise is that the listed magnification may vary unexpectedly as the patient varies their eye to lens distance, which may lead to variable performance and frustration. As the patient drifts further from the magnifier, the magnification effect will decrease. Consequently, appropriate selection of a stand magnifier depends on both visual performance as well as the patient's preferred mode of use. Training is essential to maximize the potential for success and is an integral element of LVR.

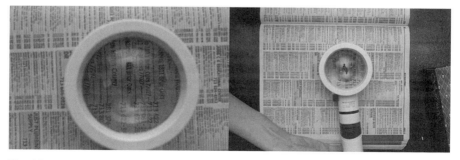

Fig. 6.3 Stand magnifier resting on a phone book to provide a virtual, enlarged image

6.5.3 Optical Devices for Distance Visual Objectives

To travel independently and view at a distance, conventional spectacle correction may not be sufficient for people with a visual impairment. Though spectacles may provide the optimal focus of the image on the retina, visual acuity may be compromised in central field loss resulting in the need for magnification. For distance objectives such as seeing street signs, bus numbers, and aisle markers in the grocery story, a hand-held telescope provides a good solution (Figure 6.4). By creating angular magnification, a telescope is able to create a larger retinal image size that may be resolved by the remaining area of functional retina.

Hand-held telescopes are typically compact and range in power from 2 to 8× magnification and are available from a number of manufacturers and distributors including Eschenbach, Optelec, Lighthouse, Walters, Specwell, and others. They are useful for quick spotting tasks and often come with a cord, so that they may be worn around the neck for easy access. Clinically prescribed telescopes are lightweight and relatively inexpensive. As the magnification increases, the field of view typically decreases (Figure 6.5). This results in a fine balance between the desired target level of acuity and the necessary field of view to quickly locate and follow the target of regard. The nomenclature for telescopes is composed of two elements: magnification and diameter of the objective lens. For a 4 × 12 telescope, the magnification is 4× and the diameter of the objective lens is 12 mm. In general, the larger the diameter of the objective lens, the larger the exit pupil and the brighter the image.

In general, the target acuity level through a telescope is 20/40. Though the actual visual demands may vary by task, the 20/40 criteria serves as a useful guideline for the initial evaluation. Elderly patients may experience difficulty in aligning and focusing the telescope, especially if they suffer from arthritis. Consequently, to maximize the probability of a good first impression, a low power (e.g., 2.5× or 2.8×) hand-held telescope may be evaluated first. Though it may not provide 20/40 acuity through the device, the relatively large field of view makes it easier to line up the telescope onto the object of regard. After pre-focusing the device, the patient is asked to line up the telescope over their better seeing eye. Despite familiarity with binoculars and other optical aids, this is not always an intuitive process. Once the

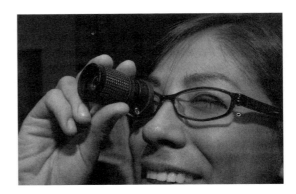

Fig. 6.4 A 4 × 12 hand-held telescope used over the right eye and spectacles to provide magnification at a distance

Fig. 6.5 The magnified image viewed through a telescope will enlarge the image at the expense of a smaller field of view

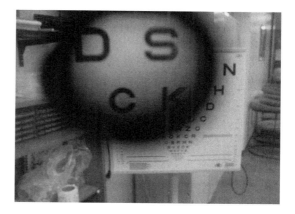

telescope is lined up on the target of regard, the patient is able to read the acuity chart to verify that they have a predictable response to magnification. For instance, a patient with 20/100 acuity would be expected to see the 20/40 line with a 2.5× hand-held telescope. This is calculated by taking the denominator of the Snellen acuity divided by the magnification of the telescope.

If the response is consistent, training with the hand-held telescope is carried out to assure that the patient is able to demonstrate the ability to focus, to spot, and to scan with the device (Figure 6.6). Training is an integral part of LVR and key to a successful outcome. Without training, the likelihood of the device ending up unused in a drawer rises significantly [24]. The amount of time required for training varies; however, a combination of in-office training and take-home exercises can optimize results.

An alternative to hand-held telescopes, bioptic telescopic spectacle (BTS) systems provide a hands-free option for distance viewing. The leading manufacturers include Designs for Vision, Inc. (Ronkonkoma, NY) and Ocutech, Inc. (Chapel

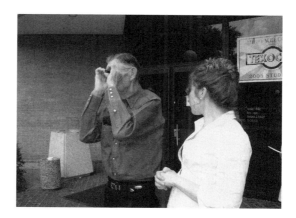

Fig. 6.6 Patient training to focus on a distant object outdoors under the guidance of a certified low-vision therapist (CLVT)

Fig. 6.7 Bioptic telescopic
spectacle illustrating the
ability to see alternately
between the carrier lens and
the telescope (courtesy of
Ocutech, Inc.)

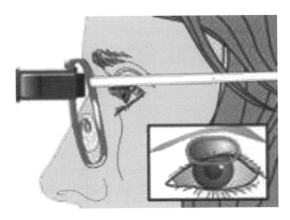

Hill, NC). BTSs are spectacle-mounted telescopes composed of two optical elements: a carrier lens with the traditional distance prescription and a telescope usually mounted in the glasses (Figure 6.7). Evolution of the technology has included
adoption of auto-focus ability in some BTS by Ocutech. BTS are particularly useful
for sporting and theater events for prolonged distance viewing. Perhaps even more
importantly, they provide some elderly visually impaired with an opportunity to
continue driving legally in over 34 States.

Driving is integral to quality of life, independent travel, maintenance of employment, and financial independence for both the normally sighted and the visually
impaired. Cessation of driving is linked to social isolation and subsequent depression [25, 26]. Regrettably, adults who lose driving privileges as a result of acquired
vision loss may experience a lowering of self-esteem and a declining level of social
status [27].

In some countries and states, a BTS may be utilized by the visually impaired to
qualify for a driver's license (Figure 6.8). The visually impaired driver spends the
majority of their time processing visual information acquired through the relatively
unobstructed view of the carrier lens and regular prescription portion of the lens.
When distance detail information is required, the user simply tilts their chin down

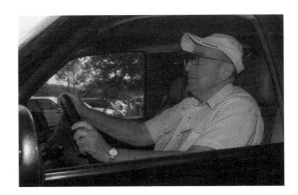

Fig. 6.8 A patient using a
bioptic telescopic spectacle
from Designs for Vision, Inc.
for driving

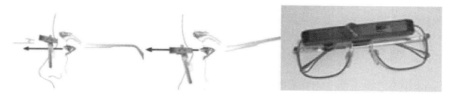

Fig. 6.9 (Right) To use the bioptic telescopic spectacle (BTS), the chin is tilted downward and the telescope is aligned in the straight-ahead position for the magnified view. (Left) A picture of the Ocutech K-mount BTS (Courtesy of Ocutech, Inc.)

slightly to align the telescope in the straight-ahead position (Figure 6.9). The magnified image is viewed briefly, and the eye is returned to the resting position through the carrier lens. The strategy is analogous to the brief look through the side or rearview mirror in a car, which is an important component of good defensive driving.

BTSs have been used to aid the visually impaired to maximize distance detail vision for tasks including driving as early as 1969 in the USA [28]. Initial experience in the USA in the 1970s raised some controversy regarding the balance between the need for detail vision and the concomitant decrease in field of view through the BTS [29–32]. Critics of BTS driving cite the decreased field of view when looking through the telescope as well as the visual field loss secondary to the ring scotoma created by the housing of the telescope itself. In addition, concern about disturbances in spatial judgment as a result of the magnified view through the BTS may lead to difficulty in accuracy of alignment. Supporters for BTS use in driving cite the improved visual acuity resulting from the magnified image through the telescope and consider proper training an essential component for successful use of the device for driving. They emphasize the very brief time spent in the telescope to access visual information as a key element to safe driving. Moreover, they argue that there are no laws prohibiting normally sighted people from driving under adverse conditions resulting in poor visibility such as heavy rain, fog, and snow. It has been suggested that poor visibility from inclement weather may have an even greater impact than that experienced by the visually impaired [27].

Driving is a complex task requiring the driver to integrate and process visual information "from both central and peripheral vision in a visually cluttered environment with little or no advance warning" [25]. Despite its complexity, crash risk comparisons have been done for handicapped versus visually handicapped drivers who score approximately the same. The accident rate per 100 drivers was 8.50 for those with neurological problems, 5.63 for those with cardiovascular impairments, and only 4.86 for those with a vision handicap [26]. Similarly, Korb found that during a 6-year period, 128 patients in Massachusetts wearing a BTS had a lower accident rate than the general driving population [28].

At the Center for Sight Enhancement at the University of Houston College of Optometry, we provide a comprehensive driving rehabilitation program that strives to maximize safety and driver confidence. On our team, the optometrist prescribes the BTS to optimize the balance between magnification, field of view, and cosmesis.

Our certified low-vision therapist conducts a training regimen with the patient to assure that they are able to quickly get in and out of the BTS, as well as spot and track with the device. The complexity of the task is gradually increased from the patient being stationary to ambulating. The next step involves the patient utilizing the device as a passenger in the car to identify a series of signs, signals, and landmarks around designated routes. Upon successful completion of this step, we collaborate with an orientation and mobility specialist, who is also a certified driving instructor, to complete a behind-the-wheel evaluation with the patient and to recommend additional training as needed. The final step involves a behind-the-wheel examination by a trooper from the Texas Department of Public Safety to verify the skills necessary to safely operate a motor vehicle. Upon successful completion of the test, the patient is eligible to receive a restricted driver's license. The emphasis on training throughout is to assure safe and effective use of the BTS during the driving task. A number of similar programs have also enjoyed successful outcomes in other states.

6.5.4 Adaptive Technology

Low-vision patients, young and old, are increasingly comfortable with technology. Closed circuit televisions (CCTVs) for electronic magnification for reading have evolved in recent years into multi-functional video magnifier systems (VMSs). These systems provide a simple method to increase the size of text, images, and maps for easier viewing. Traditionally, stand-alone VMSs consisted of a camera, moveable x-y table, and monitor. The camera provided an electronic image that could be enlarged and manipulated for display. Historically, the most common display was a CRT; however, as with computers, LCD monitors are becoming more common place. The material to be viewed is placed on an x-y table that can be moved in two dimensions to access the material displayed on the monitor (Figure 6.10).

An interesting development in recent iterations of the VMSs is the use of software to manipulate the text itself. Working like a document reader, the MyReader

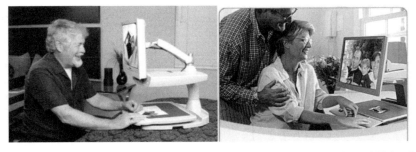

Fig. 6.10 LCD flat panels on adjustable arms. Depicted are the Merlin from Enhanced Vision (left) and ClearView from Optelec/Tiemann (right) (courtesy of Enhanced Vision and Optelec)

(HumanWare, Christchurch, New Zealand) scans a page of print into the unit, which is then able to play back the text in a variety of different presentation formats. In lieu of the x-y table to scan across a page, text may be scrolled across the monitor at varying sizes like the ticker tape on a stock channel. Similarly, text of varying size may be presented in a rapid serial visual presentation (RSVP) similar to flash cards. The primary benefit to this approach is that it minimizes the need to make accurate eye movements that are difficult to control in the presence of central blind spot.

The platforms themselves have evolved to include pocket, portable, and even wearable devices for electronic magnification and image enhancement. Thus, an increasing number of tasks may be within reach for the elderly visually impaired. To address the increasing demand, a number of manufacturers in the field have emerged including Enhanced Vision (Huntington Beach, CA), Optelec/Tiemann, Vision Technology, Inc. (St. Louis, MO), Humanware, and Freedom Scientific, among others.

In our practice, we utilize the desktop VMSs as part of our examination procedure for every patient with an interest in reading regardless of visual acuity. First, it provides diagnostic information regarding the patient's optimal magnification. Second, it permits the patient to utilize the latest adaptive technology and recognizes the potential ease with which it may meet their reading goals, whether now or at some future date. Lastly, it assures the patient that their low-vision evaluation encompasses the gamut of adaptive devices that may be of benefit to them.

From a diagnostic standpoint, we use a VMSs to provide the following information: preferred working distance from the print/screen, contrast and polarity (black on white, white on black, color combination, etc.), and enlargement ratio. One of the principal advantages of the VMSs is that the patient may sit at a more comfortable distance from the screen displaying their reading material. Given the choice between using a $5\times$ microscope at 5 cm from their eye or sitting 50 cm from a monitor, its not hard to imagine which might be the more comfortable option. Next, regardless of acuity, there are a number of conditions that benefit from the increased contrast with VMSs including glaucoma, multiple sclerosis, optic nerve atrophy, retinitis pigmentosa, and AMD, and others. Lastly, the degree of magnification or enlargement that the patient finds most comfortable on the VMSs can often provide valuable insight into the final prescriptions and highlight the need for acuity reserve for comfortable reading.

An example of where VMSs might be useful would be for a patient with 20/200 vision with AMD who is able to read 2M print at 20 cm. This corresponds to slightly larger than the large print Reader's Digest. The patient might be interested in being able to track their retirement portfolio and would like to read the stock market tables, which we assume to be about 0.5M print. To read this print, they would have to hold the stock table at about 5 cm with the appropriate correction, which might include a +20D lens ($5\times$ magnifier). However, using the VMSs, we determine that they are most comfortable sitting 50 cm from the screen, which is the same situation that they have for their computer. With white print on a black screen (reverse polarity), they appreciate the high contrast without an excess amount of light or glare. The improvement is especially noticeable when compared to the regular newspaper. To

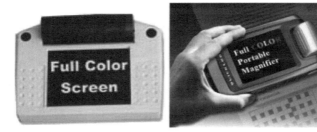

Fig. 6.11 Pocket video magnifier systems provide color, enlargement, and contrast manipulation. Compact courtesy of Optelec, Inc. (left) and QuickLook courtesy of Ash Technologies (right)

identify the optimal magnification, the patient brackets about an enlargement ratio that provides the optimal balance between legibility and field of view. The greater the magnification, the easier it is to read but the fewer the number of words that are visible on the screen at one time. Ideally, they should find a happy middle ground and slide the material on the x-y table to access print across the line. In this case, our patient enlarges the stock table size a factor of 12 on the screen, thus creating the effect of holding the stock table at 50 cm/12 or 4.2 cm away from their eye. The diagnostic information that we glean includes the importance of contrast to maximize the legibility of the print and a desire for a slightly increased acuity reserve because of the increased magnification.

Pocket VMSs have been developed using LCD displays to both magnify and enhance the image. An alternative to hand-held, illuminated, optical magnifiers, they provide a wide range of magnification along with the ability to manipulate contrast and color. Powered by rechargeable batteries, they provide their own light source and have proven to be ideal for reading tasks away from the house. This includes reading menus, labels, and magazines. A number of devices are available including the, Compact (Optelec) QuickLook (Ash Technologies, Naas, Ireland), and Pico (Telesensory, Mountain View, CA) (Figure 6.11).

Portable VMSs are larger than the pocket VMSs and typically provide a wider range of magnification, larger LCD display, and longer viewing time per battery charge. The devices may be adjusted to allow for both reading and writing. Some include a freeze frame feature to take a picture of an object of interest for more

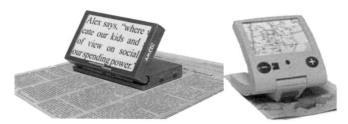

Fig. 6.12 Portable video magnifier systems have larger screens and a wider range of magnification. Shown here are the Amigo (left) and Traveller (right)

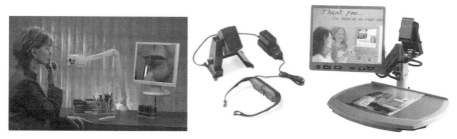

Fig. 6.13 Hybrid video magnifiers that may be used for distance and near targets provide a great deal of flexibility and independence. Devices shown here from left to right are the Acrobat and Flipper Port (courtesy of Enhanced Vision, Inc.), and the Select VMS (courtesy of Vision Technology, Inc.)

detailed review without having to keep the device on the target. Devices include the Amigo (Enhanced Vision) and Traveller (Optelec) (Figure 6.12).

Hybrid VMSs combine the ability to magnify targets at both distance and close up. Displays may be output to portable LCD panels, virtual reality goggles, or traditional computer monitors. The primary benefit is versatility in being able to direct the camera to various distances with auto-focus available to provide a clear image. Devices in this category include the Acrobat and Flipper from Enhanced Vision and the Select VMS from Vision Technology, Inc. (Figure 6.13).

In an effort to combine portability and functionality, a technology was developed to put video magnification into self-contained head-borne systems. Magnified images are displayed electronically into goggles like a virtual reality display. The Jordy II (Enhanced Vision) is an example of the device named after Engineer Geordie La Forge from the science fiction series *Star Trek: The Next Generation* (Figure 6.14). They are able to use auto-focus and zoom to enlarge objects at a distance, which make it ideal for viewing sporting events, television, and theater. Using a compact, portable control pack, patients are able to manipulate the image with variable magnification and contrast enhancement. Similarly, using an optical reading cap, the units are able to also be used for near and intermediate tasks such as reading, hand work, and activities of daily living. A desktop stand can be used to hold the Jordy II, which may be plugged into a conventional television to act as a regular desktop VMS.

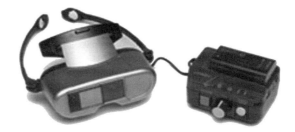

Fig. 6.14 Jordy II head-borne video magnifier system with virtual display (courtesy of Enhanced Vision, Inc.)

6.6 Future Technology

Future treatment of visual impairment utilizing bioengineering technology has made rapid advances. Foremost among the techniques being developed is the use of retinal prosthetics that integrate with existing retinal architecture. The retina is composed of a number of layers of cells that respond to light and also pre-process the signal before transmission through the optic nerve to the cortex. In the initial step, photoreceptors transduce light into chemical and electrical signals, which relay information up the pathway to ganglion cells, Mueller cells, amacrine cells, and others. In cases of retinal degeneration, photoreceptors are compromised while sparing the cells downstream. Consequently, the premise of using retinal prosthetics is to use artificially generated electrical stimulation in response to light, which may in turn drive the surviving cells downstream in the visual pathway resulting in visual perception.

The two primary approaches to date are epiretinal (on top of the retina) and subretinal (below the sensory retina) implants. The epiretinal approach uses an external camera and computer to drive a semi-conductor-based implant. The epiretinal implant consists of a series of electrodes arranged in a pattern that results in visual sensation and light response [33, 34]. Retinal and cortical activity have been demonstrated in blind patients using this method of stimulating the retina. The advantage is that the presence of ganglion cells and their axons appear sufficient to generate a response. However, as it is further downstream in the pathway, pre-processing of the signal is lost resulting in a coarser response and more limited resolution.

The subretinal approach uses an array of microphotodiodes that do not require a battery or external hardware to function. The array is only 25 µm thick and approximately 1 mm in diameter. It is designed to generate an electric current in response to light. Its location further upstream in the visual pathway, compared to the epiretinal prosthetic, increases the possibility of harnessing the inner retinal circuitry to pre-process the signal making it more similar to the natural photoreceptor response. Activation of the central visual pathway is hoped to improve the potential for better resolution [35, 36]. A device called the artificial silicon retina (ASR; Optobionics, Inc.) has been successfully implanted in patients with retinitis pigmentosa and proven to be relatively well accepted in 4 and 6 years of follow-up testing. However, interruption of nutrient flow because of the implant has shown loss of cells in cat retina over time [37, 38].

Interestingly, a secondary phenomenon has been observed with the subretinal implants, which result in improved visual function away from the location of the device. Some subjects with the implant observed improvement in function 20° from the macula and the implant resulting in motion and light detection along with improved acuity and color vision. Though the results were not sustained, there is speculation that the presence of a subretinal implant may trigger trophic factors that may promote neuronal growth and regeneration. Although exciting, the status of retinal prosthetic in the current iteration is unrealistic for the majority of elderly patients who retain significant functional vision.

Research continues to make significant strides in technology for vision restoration as well as LVR. Along with retinal prosthetics, other areas of study include gene therapy, stem cell transplantation, and modification of retinal metabolism. In neutralizing trigger factors for apoptosis (cell death) in photoreceptors, visual function may be prolonged or even preserved.

References

1. Massof RW. The measurement of vision disability. *Optom Vis Sci.* 2002;79(8):516–552.
2. Massof RW, et al. Visual disability variables. I: the importance and difficulty of activity goals for a sample of low-vision patients. *Arch Phys Med Rehabil.* 2005;86(5):946–953.
3. American Optometric Association Low Vision Rehabilitation Section Mission Statement. Available at http://www.aoa.org/x4786.xml.
4. Department of Health and Human Services. *Disability Evaluation Under Social Security.* Washington, DC: Department of Health and Human Services; 1986.
5. The Eye Diseases Prevalence Research Group. Causes and prevalence of visual impairment among adults in the United States. *Arch Ophthalmol.* 2004;122:477–485.
6. The Lighthouse Inc. *The Lighthouse National Survey on Vision Loss: the Experience, Attitudes and Knowledge of Middle-Aged and Older Americans.* New York: The Lighthouse Inc; 1995.
7. Massof RW, et al. Visual disability variables. II: the difficulty of tasks for a sample of low-vision patients. *Arch Phys Med Rehabil.* 2005;86(5):954–967.
8. Mangione CM, et al. National Eye Institute Visual Function Questionnaire Field Test Investigators. Development of the 25-item National Eye Institute Visual Function Questionnaire. *Arch Ophthalmol.* 2001;119(7):1050–1058.
9. Teunisse RJ, et al. The Charles Bonnet syndrome: a large prospective study in the Netherlands. *Br J Psychiatry.* 1995;166:254–257.
10. Burke W. The neural basis of Charles Bonnet hallucinations: a hypothesis. *J Neurol Neurosurg Psychiatry.* 2002;73;535–541.
11. Haegerstrom-Portnoy G., et al. The SKILL Card. An acuity test of reduced luminance and contrast. Smith-Kettlewell Institute Low Luminance. *Invest Ophthalmol Vis Sci.* 1997;38(1):207–218.
12. Westheimer G. Scaling of visual acuity measurement. *Arch Ophthalmol.* 1979;97:327–330.
13. Sloan, LL. New test charts for the measurement of visual acuity at far and near distances. *Am J Ophthalmol.* 1959;48:807.
14. Carter K. Chapter 6. Comprehensive Preliminary Assessments of Low vision. In: *Understanding Low Vision*, Randall T. Jose (ed.). New York: American Foundation for the Blind; 1983.
15. Whittaker SG, Lovie-Kitchin J. Visual requirements for reading. *Optom Vis Sci.* 1993;70(1):54–65.
16. Mohammed Z, Dickinson CM. The inter-relationship between magnification, field of view and contrast reserve: the effect on reading performance. *Ophthalmic Physiol Opt.* 2000;20(6):464–472.
17. Subramanian A, Pardhan S. The repeatability of MNREAD acuity charts and variability at different test distances. *Optom Vis Sci.* 2006;83(8):572–576.
18. Ahn SJ, Legge GE, Luebker A. Printed cards for measuring low-vision reading speed. *Vision Res.* 1995;35(13):1939–1944.
19. Leat SJ, Woo GC. The validity of current clinical tests of contrast sensitivity and their ability to predict reading speed in low vision. *Eye.* 1997;11(Pt. 6):893–899.
20. Weale RA. New light on old eyes. *Nature.* 1963.8;198:944–946.
21. Freed B. Refracting the low vision patient. *J Vis Rehab.* 1987;1(4):57–61.
22. Woo GC, Mah-Leung A. The term magnification. *Clin Exp Optom.* 2001;84(3):113–119.
23. DeCarlo DK, Woo S, Woo G. Chapter 36. Patients with Low Vision. In: *Borish's Clinical Refraction*, William J. Benjamin (ed.), 2nd edition. St. Louis, MO: Butterworth-Heinemann; 2007.

24. Watson G, Jose RT. A training sequence for low vision patients. *J Am Optom Assoc.* 1976;47(11):1407–1415.
25. Owsley C, McGwin G, Jr. Vision impairment and driving. *Surv Ophthalmol.* 1999; 43(6), 535–550.
26. Barron C. Bioptic telescopic spectacles for motor vehicle driving. *J Am Optom Assoc.* 1991;62(1):37–41.
27. Appel SD, Brilliant RL, Reich LN. Driving with visual impairment: facts and issues. *J Vis Rehab.* 1990;4(1):19–31.
28. Korb DR. Preparing the visually handicapped person for motor vehicle operation. *Am J Opom Arch Am Acad Optom.* 1970;47(8):619–628.
29. Fonda G. Bioptic telescopic spectacles for driving a motor vehicle. *Arch Ophthalmol.* 1974;92(4):348–349.
30. Feinbloom W. Driving with bioptic telescopic spectacles (BTS). *Am J Optom Physiol Opt.* 1977;54(1):35–42.
31. Kelleher DK. Driving with low vision. *J Vis Impair Blind.* 1979;73(9):345–350.
32. Lippmann O, Corn AL, Lewis AC. Bioptic telescopic spectacles and driving performance: a study in Texas. *J Visual Impair Blind.* 1988;82(5):182–187.
33. Humayun MS, et al. Visual perception elicited by electrical stimulation of retina in blind humans. *Arch Ophthalmol.* 1996,114:40–46.
34. Humayun MS, et al. Visual perception in a blind subject with a chronic microelectrronic retinal prosthesis. *Vision Res.* 2003,43:2573–2581.
35. Peachey NS, Chow AY. Subretinal implantation of semiconductor-based photodiodes progress and challenges. *J Rehabil Res Dev.* 1999, 36:371–376.
36. Rizzo JF III, et al. Retinal prosthesis: an encouraging first decade with major challenges ahead. *Ophthalmology.* 2001, 108:13–14.
37. Faulkner A., et al. Status of feline retina after five years of subretinal implantation with an artificial silicon retina. *Invest Ophthalmol Vis Sci.* 2005, 46, e-abstract 1518.
38. Pardue MT, et al. Immunohistochemical studies of the retina following long-term implantation with subretinal microphotodiode arrays. *Exp Eye Res.* 2001;73:333–343.

Chapter 7
Managing Hearing Loss in Older Adults

Assessment, Intervention, and Technologies for Independence and Well Being

Matthew H. Bakke, Claire M. Bernstein, Scott J. Bally, and Janet L. Pray

7.1 Overview: The Role of Hearing

Hearing plays a fundamental role in our ability to communicate with one another and provides a critical connection with our environment. The primary impact of hearing loss is on the ability to communicate with others. It is our hearing that enables us to be aware of danger sounds, such as an approaching ambulance. And it is hearing that underlies and supports our interaction with others that is such a vital part of our daily lives at home, at work, and in leisure activities. The loss of hearing, which is prevalent in older adults, can have a significant effect on all aspects of life, affecting an older adult's sense of safety, their day-to-day functioning, and in turn their participation in activities of daily life.

The impact of hearing and the loss of hearing in older adults need to be considered within the context of the myriad of biological, psychological, and social changes that are also occurring at this stage of life. For those with limited mobility, for example, hearing may take on greater importance in their daily life, providing a connection to others that might otherwise be lost. Similarly, for older adults dealing with serious illnesses, communication is a major quality of life issue. The role of hearing to sustain connection to others, foster a sense of independence, and participation in daily activities becomes paramount.

This chapter will provide a review of the key information regarding age-related hearing loss, its impact on communication, and on the psychological and social function of the older adult. We will also introduce the implications this has for the selection and use of hearing assistive technology, and will discuss the most effective means for introducing technology and training with this technology to older adults in your care.

Matthew H. Bakke

Associate Professor, Gallaudet University, Department of Hearing, Speech and Language Sciences, Director, Rehabilitation Engineering Research Center (RERC) on Hearing Enhancement, 800 Florida Avenue, NE, MTB 116, Washington, DC 20002
e-mail: matthew.bakke@gallaudet.edu

From: *Aging Medicine, Eldercare Technology for Clinical Practitioners,*
Edited by: M. Alwan and R. Felder © Humana Press, Totowa, NJ

From the perspective of a professional working with older adults, any professional working with an older adult needs to be mindful of the prevalence of hearing loss in this population and its impact on communication. One of the most immediate practical issues professionals may face is dealing with older adults who have a hearing loss but are not wearing amplification. In fact, while the prevalence of hearing loss is approximately 40–45% for adults 65 years of age and older, only 20% of these older adults obtains hearing aids [1]. In light of this, the client may not understand the information, recommendations, directions, or counseling that is part and parcel of your professional interaction with the client.

In addition to making a referral to an audiologist for a hearing evaluation and follow-up, there are some easy-to-use hearing assistive technologies that can help facilitate the critical communication that is needed from the outset between you and your client. A simple, practical solution to assist your interactions with a client would be to have a personal hearing technology device available to use for one-to-one communication. Furthermore, there are many older adults already using amplification who may still be experiencing difficulty understanding speech, particularly if the listening environment has background noise. There are some very helpful tips for communicating with an older adult with hearing loss that could make communication easier with your client that you may want to consider. An example of such tips can be found on the Elder Care Online website, http://www.ec-online.net/Knowledge/Articles/communication.html. The importance and role of both personal and other assistive listening technologies, along with communication strategies to help both the professional and the older adult with hearing loss, is described in detail in Section 7.9.2.

7.2 Prevalence and Demographics of Hearing Loss in Older Adults

Hearing loss is currently the third most common chronic condition, after hypertension and arthritis, and the primary sensory disorder among older adults [2]. According to the US Census, 28 million Americans have significant hearing loss, which is considered to be that which interferes with successful communication. The prevalence of hearing loss is especially great among elderly people; six times more prevalent for persons 75 years and older than for those aged 18–44 years [3]. A review of the US Census Bureau data on the prevalence of disability among individuals 15 years and older reveals that the estimated prevalence of "difficulty hearing conversation" increases dramatically from 2.3% in those 25–64 years of age to 12.3% in those 65 years and older [4].

As the baby boomers, born between 1945 and 1962 reach maturity, the incidence of hearing loss is certain to increase dramatically. In 1991, 31.7 million adults were 65 years or older, with a projection of 52 million by 2020, and 70 million by 2040 [5, 6]. A disproportionate number of individuals over the age of 60 years experience hearing loss given the effects of greater longevity and increased environmental noise; both may be considered as the result of presbycusis. It is anticipated that hearing loss will affect 26% of those aged 65–74 years, 36% between 75 and 84 years, and approximately 50% of individuals who are 85 years and older [7]. The latter is the fastest growing segment of the US population and is expected to triple between 2000 and 2040 [6]. Three independent studies provide evidence that 70–80% of older adults who are institutionalized have measurable hearing loss, the loss being greater with advancing age [8–10]. Given the effect of hearing loss on communication, addressing the needs of older adults with hearing loss must take a high priority for any professional working with this population.

Changing demographics that influence this population also include population shifts, including trends toward dispersed families and changing family roles. Older adults tend to gravitate toward specific geographic areas (e.g., Florida, Arizona, New York) and are often not living near their families. Additionally, although there is a perception that the majority of older adults are institutionalized, in fact the majority live independently, 95% as opposed to 5% [11]. That being said, this varies by age such that for adults aged 65–74 years, approximately 3% reside in a nursing home, compared with 22% of those 85 years of age and older (11). This has a significant impact on the support systems and health care delivery for older adults when they are faced with adversity, and hearing loss in particular.

7.3 Characteristics of Hearing Loss

7.3.1 Degrees of Hearing Loss

The descriptors used to describe the hearing loss of an older adult relates to both hearing thresholds (pure tone average or PTA) and aural communication functioning. Table 7.1 presents commonly accepted threshold ranges for degree of hearing loss established by Goodman [12] and modified by Clark [13] as well as implications for speech understanding and social functioning.

It is important to note that most hearing losses are not limited to a specific degree of loss. Many older adults have a range of hearing loss such as mild to moderate, or moderate to profound. In such cases, the above descriptors must be interpreted on a case by case basis.

7.3.2 Types of Hearing Loss: (Conductive, Sensorineural, Mixed)

The way in which hearing loss is managed is dependent on the types of hearing loss identified. Conductive hearing loss refers to conditions in the outer or middle ear, which impede the transmission of sound. Examples include a middle ear infection, impacted wax, a ruptured ear drum, to name a few. This type of hearing loss lends itself to medical and/or surgical intervention, and is typically seen as reversible.

Sensorineural hearing loss refers to conditions in the inner ear (cochlea) or along the nerve that sends the acoustic information to the brain. Among the most common causes are aging, noise exposure, ototoxic drugs, and genetic factors. Typically,

Table 7.1 Degrees of Hearing Loss

Mild hearing loss (26–40 dB)	Even mild hearing loss may have significant impact on communication; there may be difficulty hearing quiet speech, especially with background noise such as music or multiple conversations. Some speech sounds may be distorted or faint. However, speechreading may supplement receptive understanding
Moderate hearing loss (41–55 dB)	Frequent difficulties with conversational speech. Considerable difficulty following conversation with competing signals (e.g., spouse speaking and football game on TV). Amplification may provide significant improvement in receptive ability. Hearing aids may provide access to most speech sounds and communication in quiet, while other assistive hearing technology (e.g., FM systems) may provide access even with competing noise. Speechreading skills may supplement receptive understanding
Moderately severe hearing loss (56–70 dB)	Frequent difficulties even with loud speech. Significant difficulty following any conversation, especially when compounded by competing signals. Most speech sounds are inaccessible during normal conversation. Hearing aids may provide access to most speech sounds and communication in quiet, whereas other assistive hearing technologies are needed to provide access in the presence of competing noise. Access to visual information (speechreading) becomes more critical for successful communication
Severe hearing loss (71–90 dB)	Inability to understand even loud speech. Unable to follow conversations. Speech sounds are inaccessible during normal conversation, even in optimum listening environment. Hearing aids enable access for sound detection, although most speech sounds cannot be discriminated or identified. Both speechreading and hearing assistive technology are critical for providing linguistic cues such as suprasegmentals (e.g., pitch, loudness, rhythm). Cochlear implants may be considered, whereas others may choose American sign language (ASL) or other signed languages for communication
Profound hearing loss (91 to 110+ dB)	Inability to detect even loud speech and important environmental sounds (e.g., ambulances, car horns, growling dogs). Hearing aids provide limited assistance for sound awareness; speech sounds cannot be identified. Both speechreading and hearing assistive technology are critical for providing linguistic cues such as suprasegmentals (e.g. pitch, loudness, rhythm). Cochlear implants should be considered, while others may choose ASL or other signed languages for communication

sensorineural hearing loss cannot be remediated medically or surgically. However, this type of hearing loss may be managed with hearing aids and other hearing assistive technologies, and the use of communication strategies. For those without residual hearing, the use of sign language may be a viable alternative for communication within limited contexts.

On occasion, an individual may sustain a mixed hearing loss, wherein a conductive hearing loss occurs in combination with a sensorineural hearing loss. For example, an individual with a genetic hearing loss may have an ear infection that would further reduce their hearing thresholds. In these situations, the conductive component would be treated medically.

7.3.3 Nature of Hearing Loss

The most critical factor affecting communication may be the nature of the hearing loss. Simply stated, some individuals experience a loss of loudness, whereas others experience a lack of clarity. A loss of loudness reflects a loss of hearing sensitivity, meaning that sounds must be louder in order for them to be heard. This type of hearing loss responds well to amplification. A lack of clarity, or discrimination ability, suggests that although sounds may be loud enough they are not clear enough to identify. Providing amplification has limited effectiveness in that sounds are louder but usually not clearer. More recent hearing aids are able to equalize sound intensity across frequencies thereby giving the perception of greater clarity and do in fact increase understanding of receptive communication. This is discussed in greater depth in the section 6 entitled *Age-Related Changes to the Inner Ear: Impact on Communication and Implications for Technology Assessment and Use*.

7.3.4 Characteristics of Age-Related Hearing Loss

The term presbycusis is used to describe age-related hearing loss. Presbycusis is a complex of hearing loss associated with aging, combined with a decrease in speech understanding. Most older adults experience a gradual onset of hearing loss, which is typically mild to moderate in degree. The type of hearing loss is sensorineural because of damage to the inner ear and central auditory nervous system. In terms of the nature of the hearing loss, presbycusis is progressive, bilateral and symmetrical (i.e., both ears affected equally), and irreversible. The greatest loss of hearing sensitivity is found in the higher frequency range, with noted difficulty understanding speech, particularly rapid speech and speech in noise.

Although presbycusis affects both men and women, it typically begins at an earlier age for men, with hearing declining by age 30 years [14, 15]. The pattern of hearing loss is seen as a sharp decrease in hearing for the high frequencies. Typically, vowel information and voicing is carried in the lower frequencies, whereas consonants, which provide the clarity of speech, are carried in the higher frequencies. Hearing continues to decline over the decades for men; average hearing thresholds for men between the ages of 65 and 89 years reflect an average 10 decibel decrement per decade across the high frequency range [14].

Data from the Baltimore Longitudinal Study [15] indicate that women show a greater loss in low frequency sensitivity, with a decline in hearing accelerating between ages 40 and 50 years. The earlier onset of hearing loss in men, combined with a greater loss in high-frequency sensitivity, is generally attributed to greater noise exposure related to occupational and/or military exposure.

7.3.5 Other Symptoms of Auditory Disorders

7.3.5.1 Tinnitus

Tinnitus is described by the American Tinnitus Association as "the perception of sound in the ears or head where no external source is present" [16]. Although population-based estimates of the prevalence of tinnitus in the USA are difficult to find, current estimates based on the National Health Interview Survey [17] indicate that 2.98% of all Americans have chronic tinnitus. The prevalence of tinnitus increases with increasing age so that 5.96% report chronic tinnitus between the ages of 45 and 64 years, and 8.77% over 65 years. Applying these prevalence estimates to the 2000 census data [18] indicates that over 3 million people over the age of 65 years and over 8 million Americans of all ages experience chronic tinnitus [19].

The causes of tinnitus are not well understood and are multiple. It is commonly associated with hearing loss, and there are both cochlear and neural hypotheses about the underlying physiological mechanisms [19, 20]. Because many disease conditions (such as vascular disease, middle-ear disease, diabetes among others) are associated with tinnitus, it is important to consider tinnitus as a clinical sign when performing diagnostic procedures, and it is recommended that all tinnitus patients should be referred to an otologist [19, 21]. Tinnitus can affect those who experience it differently and with varying degrees of severity, including such effects as loss of sleep, irritability, weariness, distractibility, interference with work or social activities, and enjoyment [22]. Sleep problems are a particularly important issue to address with tinnitus patients. More than 70% of the sample of patients in the Tinnitus Data Registry, a research database maintained by the Oregon Hearing Research Center, reported sleep disturbances resulting from tinnitus [22]. However, many people have tinnitus that is not reported, probably because they do not consider it to have enough impact on their everyday lives. About 80% of those with chronic tinnitus do not seek treatment for their tinnitus [19].

Because its manifestations and severity are so variable, treatment of tinnitus proves to be a difficult task. Many approaches have been recommended, including the use of amplification, tinnitus maskers, counseling, psychological treatments, pharmacological approaches, tinnitus-retraining therapy (TRT), electrical stimulation, temporomandibular joint (TMJ) treatment, and other alternative treatments such as nutritional supplements and acupuncture [19, 23]. However, at this time, there is not a good body of well-controlled research to support decisions about clinical practice, and a consensus will be necessary in the future in order to standardize research and clinical practice in the field.

7.3.5.2 Balance Disorders and Older Adults

The vestibular system plays a key role in balance. Housed within the inner ear, the vestibular system is made up of three components—the semicircular canals, the utricle, and the saccule. Sensory hair cells in the vestibular system are activated by the movement of this inner ear fluid (i.e., endolymph) in response to movement and position of the body. When the head moves, these hair cells send impulses to the brain through the vestibular part of the acoustic nerve.

Dizziness is the most common complaint of patients aged 75 years or older. Balance disorders secondary to dizziness are responsible for over one-third of falls in older adults [24]. Moreover, balance disorders place older adults at risk for injuries, with falls often resulting in functional disability, and representing the leading cause of accidental death in adults 75 years and older [25]. The diagnosis and management of balance disorders, and particularly the assessment of risk for falls, is of paramount importance with older adults.

Balance function is dependent upon the integrity of the visual system, somatosensory system, the central nervous system, as well as the vestibular system. A constellation of factors, including muscle strength, joint mobility, changes in vision, loss of sensation in the feet, and cardiovascular factors, all may impact the sense of stability and equilibrium. Medications and drug interactions can also contribute to symptoms of unsteadiness. Another issue to consider with older adults is the prevalence of benign paroxysmal positional vertigo (BPPV). BPPV is a type of dizziness caused by abnormal reaction of the balance organ to certain head movements. When crystals that normally occur in the inner ear are displaced into the semicircular canals, they can stimulate the balance nerve inappropriately.

A balance assessment protocol with an older population, performed by an audiologist, needs to go beyond electronystagmography (ENG) testing. Older adults require a more comprehensive evaluation including, but not limited to, rotational tests and computerized posturography with static and dynamic balance testing, sensory stimulation testing, neurologic exam, along with assessment of range of motion, muscle strength, and peripheral neuropathy. It is often the case that the presence of one problem may not represent the complete picture in an older individual. Audiologists play a key role in making recommendations for rehabilitation and further evaluation. Current treatment programs of vestibular rehabilitation, while not removing symptoms of unsteadiness, offer older adults increased confidence in their mobility and lessen the functional impact of the balance disorder.

Given the complexity of balance disorders in older adults, a multidisciplinary approach is critical. Ideally, this would involve the combined expertise of audiologists, otolaryngologists, neurotologists, ophthalmologists, neurologists, physical and occupational therapists, and specialists in geriatric medicine. The reader is directed to Chapter 8 for a comprehensive review of balance disorders in older adults.

7.4 Causes and Prevention of Age-Related Hearing Loss

The study of age-related hearing loss has been approached from a variety of perspectives that include epidemiological studies, animal models, and post-mortem temporal bone studies. The key question under investigation has been whether age-related hearing loss is solely a function of aging, genetics, the result of environmental effects, notably noise exposure, or a combination of these factors.

Epidemiologic studies document decrease in hearing with advancing age, citing age as the most important risk factor associated with hearing loss [14, 26, 27]. Longitudinal research conducted by Gates and Cooper [28], Brant et al. [29], and Cruickshanks et al. [30] has identified additional risk factors that may account for some of the age-related changes in hearing sensitivity. These risk factors include noise exposure, smoking, systolic blood pressure, cardiovascular disease, ototoxic medications, and family history of hearing impairment. These additional risk factors are of particular interest because appropriate clinical management, such as improved control over systolic blood pressure, may in turn serve to reduce the extent of hearing loss.

The classic work of Schuknecht and Gacek [31] involved temporal bone studies that yielded classification of presbycusis based on an analysis of pathologic changes. The defining criteria for each type of presbycusis was determined by histopathological changes observed in outer hair cells, inner hair cells, the stria vascularis, and in neuronal loss based on distance from the base of the cochlea. Schuknecht and Gacek [31] found that it was not possible to differentiate histological changes resulting from aging from those caused by noise or ototoxicity, particularly for the sensory type of presbycusis.

A comprehensive review by Henderson et al. [32] on the role of oxidative stress in noise-induced hearing loss gives further evidence of the similarities in cochlear pathology and audiologic changes for hearing losses that result from noise, ototoxic drugs, and aging. Findings from studies on ototoxic drugs [33], noise exposure [34], and antioxidants and aging [35] all point to a common underlying process involving the role of oxidative stress (i.e., free radical damage at the cellular level) and damage to the cochlea.

The role of genetics in age-related hearing loss has come to the forefront in recent years. Family history of hearing loss has taken on greater importance in the management of presbycusis. Gates et al. [36], in a large study of older adults and their children, found that having a parent with age-related hearing loss increases the risk of hearing loss, indicating a significant genetic link for presbycusis. An animal model of age-related hearing loss has also been used to look at the role of genetics and hearing loss. Working with a mouse model, the location of a single gene that influences age-related hearing loss has been identified [37]. The age-related hearing loss gene, named *AHL*, is thought to mediate a decrease in protective enzymes, causing an increase in the level of oxidative stress, which is turn leads to auditory degeneration. Additional studies have also found an interaction between the age-related hearing loss gene and greater susceptibility to noise-induced hearing loss [38]. Although this research has been carried out in mice, if it turns out to hold true for people, there are significant implications for counseling. Specifically, if there is a genetic predisposition to hearing loss, it is crucial to counsel our patients to limit their noise exposure and use hearing protection.

Overall, studies from various perspectives all indicate that age-related hearing loss is a function of numerous factors including genetics, noise, and ototoxic exposure, along with changes occurring because of aging in the auditory system. The interaction of these factors leads to the clinical recommendation of eliminating and/or reducing exposure to noise and ototoxic drugs to minimize the additional impact it may have on the hearing of an older adult. Additional risk factors, such as high blood pressure and smoking, and cardiovascular status, also have a bearing on the extent of hearing loss and appropriate management can benefit an older adult's hearing as well as their health in general. Finally, given the similarities in cochlear pathology and audiologic changes observed for hearing loss associated with aging, ototoxicity, and noise, a convergence of new clinical interventions to address all of these types of hearing losses may lie ahead.

7.5 Age-Related Changes in the Auditory System and Implications for Technology Assessment and Use

This section addresses the key anatomical and physiological changes occurring in the auditory system of older adults and the functional implications of these changes. Age-related changes in the auditory system can have a direct and significant impact on hearing and, in turn, communication function. These changes may also directly impact assessment along with the selection and use of hearing technology. For this reason, it is important to understand what is occurring with age and how it affects clinical practice.

There are many systemic changes that occur because of the aging process that manifests itself in the auditory system as well. These include, but are not limited to, changes in connective tissue, skin, muscle, bone, along with concomitant changes in the cardiovascular, respiratory, and nervous system. With this framework in mind, we will review age-related changes occurring along the auditory system, beginning with the outer ear, progressing through the middle and inner ear, then along the auditory nerve and up through the central auditory nervous system. As these changes are described, we will highlight how they may affect testing, impact the communication capabilities of an older adult, or affect the selection of hearing technology and/or its use.

7.5.1 Outer Ear

The outer ear comprises the pinna, which collects and localizes sounds, and includes the s-shaped ear canal that sends sounds to the eardrum, referred to as the tympanic membrane. Age-related changes to the outer ear include the degeneration of elastic fibers and decrease in collagen, which occurs systemically to connective tissue throughout the body. These changes, in turn, result in a loss of elasticity and strength of the outer ear and are responsible for the presence of collapsed canals, with a prevalence as high as 30–40% in the older population [39]. Collapsed canals pose difficulties for testing and require special consideration when hearing aids and other assistive hearing technologies are considered for fitting with an older adult. Novak [40] points out that an older adult may not be able to wear a particular style of hearing aid, or may reject the technology entirely if special approaches are not taken to ensure that soreness or irritation will not result from placement in a collapsed ear canal.

Another age-related change of considerable significance is the noted decline in the secretory ability of the sebaceous and cerumenous glands. Instead of the normal process whereby cerumen, known as ear wax, is naturally removed from the ear (i.e., epithelial migration), what occurs instead is the development of hard and impacted cerumen; this has far reaching implications. In and of itself, impacted cerumen can cause a mild-to-moderate degree of hearing loss. Although this hearing loss is reversible once cerumen is removed, it is often superimposed on an existing sensorineural hearing loss that is not reversible, thus compounding the communication difficulties faced by an older adult. Impacted cerumen may also preclude many diagnostic tests and measures that are needed to help fit an older adult with hearing technology. This is a very frequent occurrence in the older population, with estimates running as high as 35% [41]. As such, the management of impacted cerumen is critical to successful assessment and intervention programs.

In addition, older adults typically present with less fat in the ear canal and increased length of the hair follicles, which is turn leads to dry skin that is prone to trauma and breakdown. This can affect the management of cerumen removal and make the ear canal more sensitive in the bony portion (e.g., the inner third of the canal, which is closest to the tympanic membrane) to the placement of devices such as ear molds, hearing aids, or other hearing technology that need to be fit in the canal. This problem is magnified for those older adults who have coexisting medical conditions such as diabetes or are immuno-compromised, where extreme care must be taken in the removal of impacted cerumen to ensure that no further sequelae occur.

7.5.2 Middle Ear

The middle ear, which begins at the tympanic membrane, is an air-filled space consisting of three small bones that send the sound from the tympanic membrane, more commonly known as the eardrum, to the inner ear. The eustachian tube, which connects the middle ear to the nasopharynx, provides ventilation and air pressure equalization in the middle ear space. Although the tympanic membrane is found to become stiffer, thinner, and less vascular with aging, the impact of these changes on both testing and management remains limited. The ossicular chain, however, consisting of the malleus, incus, and stapes bones, is affected by the systemic changes that occur to bones and joints throughout the body. Specifically, age-related changes to the middle ear include ossification of the bones and calcification of the joints in the middle ear, whereby the transmission of sound becomes less efficient. This problem is of greatest concern for those older adults who have severe forms of arthritis. These older adults present not only with hearing loss but coexisting dexterity issues that must be considered in the selection, fitting, and use of any hearing technology.

Perhaps the most significant age-related change impacting the middle ear is found with the eustachian tube. The eustachian tube connects the middle ear with the nasopharynx, providing equalization of ear pressure on both sides of the tympanic membrane; opening of the tube is most noticeable during swallowing and yawning. With aging, calcification of the cartilaginous support is observed along with atrophy of the musculature that supports the eustachian tube. This, in turn, interferes with opening of the tube, making the ear more prone to infection. Of all middle ear disorders, older adults are most prone to developing an infectious disease of the middle ear. Changes in muscle function of the eustachian tube with age, combined with a tendency of older adults to develop complications following upper respiratory infections, and a less efficient immune system, all contribute to a greater susceptibility for older adults to develop an infectious disease of the middle ear. When this occurs, medical management is needed to ensure that the infection is treated promptly, and to limit any disruption of hearing technology use that may ensue because of an active middle ear infection.

7.5.3 Inner Ear

The inner ear, which is buried deep in the bones of the skull, consists of the cochlea, the balance system, and the auditory nerve. The function of the cochlea is to interpret the different frequencies, or pitches, of sounds we hear. The sound is then transmitted to the brain by way of the auditory nerve.

7.5.3.1 Cochlea

The cochlea is the structure that is the most susceptible to age-related changes. The most salient age-related change found in the cochlea is the loss of sensory hair cells. Because hair cells are highly differentiated cells, this means that once their function is set, they no longer reproduce. The impact of this is important because once these hair cells are lost they cannot be replaced.

The cochlea comprises inner and outer hair cells, both of which degenerate with age. It should be noted that this degeneration can occur independently. In all, sensory hair cell loss is the rule among older adults, with the greatest loss in people over the age of 70 years. The outer hair cells have been found to be the most vulnerable and account for the typical decline in hearing with age. Furthermore, the greatest loss of hair cells is found at the base of the cochlea, which is the entrance to the organ of hearing, and produces the pattern of high-frequency hearing loss that typifies presbycusis [42].

7.5.3.2 Auditory Nerve

The auditory nerve links the sensory hair cells of the cochlea to the brainstem. A relationship has been found between age and the loss of ganglion cells in the auditory nerve. Young adults typically possess 30–40,000 ganglion cells. This neuronal population decreases over the decades such that between the ages of 50–70 years there are approximately 25,000 ganglion cells remaining. By age 80 years, the neuronal population has decreased to below 20,000 [43, 44].

The loss of ganglion cells is greatest near the base of the cochlea, yet remains independent of sensory cell loss. When the loss of ganglion cells near the base of the cochlea exceeds 50%, it is associated with high-frequency hearing loss. There are conflicting reports on the functional implications resulting from the loss of ganglion cells. There are some who state that significant ganglion cell loss results in poor speech recognition and others who claim that the loss of ganglion cells, while resulting in a high-frequency hearing loss, does not compromise the speech recognition ability of an older adult [43, 45]. This issue has important ramifications for the provision of rehabilitative services, hearing technology, and counseling.

7.6 Age-Related Changes to the Inner Ear: Impact on Communication and Implications for Technology Assessment and Use

The major functional implication of age-related changes to the cochlea and the auditory nerve is a high-frequency sensorineural hearing loss in both ears. In practical terms, this means that the loss of hearing is a result of age-related changes in the cochlea and/or the auditory nerve. Furthermore, damage to the hair cells and/or the auditory nerve is found at the location closest to the base of the cochlea, producing a high-frequency hearing loss. Not only is there a loss in the intensity, or loudness, of speech, but the high frequencies carry the consonant information, which is critical for determining exactly what was said. In and of itself, a sensorineural hearing loss results in decreased hearing thresholds, reduced frequency, and temporal discrimination, all of which impact auditory processing abilities, and ultimately impair communication.

Several theories have been posited to account for the significant difficulty with speech understanding that is the hallmark of presbycusis. Briefly, one perspective attributes the difficulty understanding speech to changes occurring primarily in the periphery, i.e., damage to the cochlea resulting in loss of audibility of high-frequency information and/or distortion caused by problems with temporal or intensity discrimination [46]. Another hypothesis identifies cognitive deficits, including slower processing and increased cognitive demands (e.g., short-term memory problems) as the reason behind speech recognition difficulties. Research by Bellis and Wilbur [47] attributes changes occurring with the transfer of information from one hemisphere to the other that in turn leads to problems with auditory processing. Yet another view is that changes occurring along the central auditory pathway are responsible for the difficulties in speech comprehension observed with older adults

[48, 49]. The most recent consensus [50] recognizes the role of peripheral hearing loss in relation to the speech recognition difficulties experienced by an older adult, but also attributes a portion of the difficulties to age-related declines in cognitive abilities and changes in central auditory processing abilities. With this understanding as background, it is critical that all approaches to rehabilitation and hearing technology address the unique speech recognition problems that older adults face.

The greatest consequence of hearing loss in an older adult is the impact it places on communication. Hearing loss associated with aging results in difficulty understanding speech in noise, speech under reverberant, and at times even in quiet, conditions. It is important to understand that beyond a loss of loudness that is associated with decreased hearing thresholds, there is also a reduced ability to process auditory information associated with aging that becomes apparent for older adults as the listening condition becomes more difficult. While an older adult may communicate well in a one-to-one situation, they typically experience difficulty listening to rapid speech, speakers with accents, and when listening to speech when visual cues are not available.

Gordon-Salant [51] provides an excellent review of speech understanding performance of older adults identifying the influential factors that contribute to communication problems of older adults. In addition to hearing loss, Gordon-Salant highlights the key role that temporal processing (i.e. ability to process rapidly changing auditory information) and cognitive changes play in the speech understanding performance of older adults. Problems with temporal processing are responsible for many of the performance difficulties older adults exhibit with rapid speech and speakers with accents. In terms of cognitive changes, Wingfield and Tun [52] and Gordon-Salant and Fitzgibbons [53] point to the overall slowing of processing associated with aging to account for speech understanding difficulties. This was especially evident when contextual information was not available (e.g. comprehension of words as opposed to sentence material). Taken from a different perspective, the use of contextual cues may help overcome some of the difficulties with understanding speech that older adults encounter.

Difficulty understanding speech in noise, which is an almost universal complaint among older adults, presents a significant challenge to hearing rehabilitation. Of all the hearing technologies that are currently available, recommendations are almost exclusively limited to hearing aids. Hearing aids can help older adults with hearing loss compensate for some of their difficulties, particularly understanding speech in quiet, and at times, in noise. The latest generation of hearing aids, i.e. digital aids, have advanced signal processing capabilities that offer significant advantages in improving speech understanding. The advent of certain recent special features on hearing aids, notably directional microphones, have been shown to improve the signal-to-noise ratio, reducing noise from behind or to the sides, which yield significant improvement in understanding of speech in noise for an older adult [54].

While digital hearing aids with directional microphones have made inroads for technological solutions to the key difficulty of understanding speech in noise, there are other technologies and interventions that are less frequently utilized that should be considered as well. Assistive listening technology, either in addition to hearing aids or instead of amplification, can help overcome many of the difficulties older adults experience in adverse listening situations. For example, FM technology offers a technology solution whereby both distance and noise can be overcome. Specifically, a microphone is worn by the speaker and the speech is transmitted by a radio frequency signal sent directly to the person as part of their hearing aid or as a separate receiver. This type of assistive listening technology provides significant improvement in the signal to noise ratio, allowing the older adult to understand the speaker, overcoming distance and/or surrounding noise.

With the availability of this kind of technology, there is significant improvement in speech understanding. The improvement in communication abilities can in turn offer an older adult greater independence and participation in social situations. In spite of the reported improvement in communication skills, clinical research points to a reluctance of older adults to use this technology [55]. There is sometimes a stigma associated with its use, and the individual may find it difficult to assert their listening needs to others. For this reason, there is a great need for training and counseling to help facilitate the use of this technology that can overcome communication problems. Some innovative new approaches, e.g. the role of peer mentors which is discussed in detail later in this chapter, and extensive counseling may be key to facilitate the adaptation, function, and independence of the older adult with hearing loss.

In addition to difficulty understanding speech in noise, hearing rehabilitation with older adults also needs to address their difficulty with rapid speech, listening to speakers with accents, and listening to speech when visual cues are not available. A combination of technology and rehabilitative approaches may be needed. Gordon-Salant [51] highlights two major technological developments that address this including signal processing strategies in digital hearing aids that alter the duration of speech segments, and a new device developed in Japan that enables the user to select the rate that speech will be presented at. Both of these technological solutions seem to be promising approaches to the problems with rapid speech experienced by older adults.

Focusing on the interaction of cognitive changes and speech understanding of older adults, the concept of working memory capacity described by Gatehouse et al [56] offers insight into differences in cognitive skills and their effect on speech recognition performance. Gatehouse suggests that it is important to consider these cognitive factors when hearing technology is selected. Pichora-Fuller and Singh [57] call our attention to some of the latest research on brain plasticity and the interactions of auditory and cognitive processing. The most immediate implications for clinical practice call for integrating training and rehabilitation along with hearing technology itself in order to promote brain reorganization and improve auditory functioning.

7.6.1 Central Auditory Nervous System

The central auditory nervous system deals with the transmission of sound beyond the auditory nerve, along the pathway that includes the brainstem and ends in the auditory cortex in the brain. Age-related changes that have been reported in the central auditory nervous system include the overall loss of neurons, a decrease in the size and density of neurons, and the disappearance or diminution of dendrites [42]. Some report that the neurons do not decrease in number but do evidence degeneration. Age-related changes in the central auditory nervous system have been found to be highly variable. The most significant functional implication of changes in the central auditory nervous system is an overall slowing of central processing. Not surprisingly, this in turn impacts the ability of an older adult to follow and understand conversation. This difficulty is observed even without the presence of a peripheral hearing loss, and is much greater when a hearing loss is present as well.

7.6.1.1 Auditory Processing Disorders

Martin and Jerger [50] provide a comprehensive review of the literature in this area. They cite evidence from many studies that substantiates the claim that speech understanding problems of older adults result in part from central auditory processing disorders. Difficulties observed with understanding speech become most apparent when the older adult is dealing with rapid speech, speech where there are many talkers, or in the presence of background noise. Independent of peripheral hearing loss, a decline in central auditory abilities is thought to be responsible for some of the problems with temporal processing, and consequently understanding speech that have been observed with older adults.

Age-related changes in central auditory processing have been noted in studies looking at dichotic listening abilities of older adults. In these studies the person listens to signals, typically words or digits, presented at the same time to both ears. Dichotic listening tasks are considered markers of interhemispheric processing and cooperation. It should be kept in mind that normal hemispheric asymmetry, corresponding to left hemisphere dominance and favoring the right ear, is involved in the processing of language. For older listeners a pronounced "left-ear disadvantage," that increases as the listening environment becomes more difficult has been found for speech material. This asymmetry has been observed to increase with age. Less efficient interhemispheric transfer of information is thought to contribute to the auditory processing problems of older adults Bellis and Wilbur [47, 58].

7.6.1.2 Implications for Amplification and Use of Assistive Listening Technology

Important considerations regarding both amplification and assistive listening technology are raised by Martin and Jerger [50] based on a review of the literature on aging and central auditory processing. With respect to amplification, it remains controversial whether an older adult with central auditory processing difficulties should be fit with one or two hearing aids. Although the advantages of binaural amplification are well-established [59], there are times when the introduction of binaural aids contributes additional interference and therefore adds to the processing difficulties of an older adult rather than reducing them [60]. This may be particularly true for speech understanding in challenging listening environments such as those with a good deal of background noise or reverberation. Understanding the role of central auditory factors may be key to the success of amplification with older adults.

Furthermore, although amplification provides greater access to sound, it cannot compensate for temporal processing problems associated with the central auditory system of older adults. As such, the value of assistive listening technology in addition to amplification is underscored. In particular, assistive listening technology that employs remote microphones to overcome the problems of noise and distance may offer an excellent option for older adults to help overcome the difficulties posed by hearing loss associated with aging. At the same time, the actual use of this technology with remote microphones (i.e., primarily FM systems) by older adults has been found to be a more complex process, requiring a great deal of training, counseling, and coaching in order for it to be successful [61, 62]. The training and counseling component may be as critical to successful use as the technology itself.

7.6.2 Cognitive Function

Some significant issues may influence both the accurate diagnosis of hearing loss and the potential for an individual to make successful adaptation. How an individual is affected by hearing loss is influenced by three cognitive components: what they know about hearing loss, how they perceive hearing loss, and how they problem-solve to cope with the effects of hearing loss. Clearly, better cognitive functioning enables an individual to adapt to hearing loss more successfully. The incidence of dementia in older adults over the age of 65 years has been reported to be 15%; this figure jumps to 50% for individuals over the age of 80 years [11].

7.6.2.1 Hearing Loss and Dementia

Russell and Burns [63] define senile dementia as "an acquired global impairment involving loss of intellectual function and other cognitive skills that is sufficient to interfere with social or occupational function." Criteria for dementia noted by Abrams et al. [11] include impairment in abstract thinking, as well as judgment in planning, and personality changes. The effects of hearing loss in aging may be similarly defined as a sensory impairment that is sufficient to interfere with social or occupational function and the criteria may also have parallels. It is not surprising, therefore, that differentiating between the effects of the two may be problematic. To further complicate the issue, test design for assessment in these two areas does not always clearly differentiate between the effects of hearing loss and dementia.

An association has been noted between greater degrees of hearing loss and the presence of dementia [64]. This has major implications for both diagnosis and intervention. It should also be noted that there is an increased prevalence of central auditory processing problems among older adults with dementia, increasing the complexity of working with this population.

7.6.2.2 Professional Implications

Misdiagnosis of Dementia

Given overlapping symptomatology of dementia and hearing loss, it is recommended that the client use their own hearing aids to maximize auditory input during cognitive testing. In the event that clients do not have amplification, professionals are encouraged to employ personal hearing devices such as a pocket talker during testing. For the same reason, the greatest caution should be used when interpreting the results of a differential diagnosis. If the client has a known hearing loss and amplified hearing still limits his/her understanding, results of cognitive testing may be suspect. An additional consideration is the influence of some medications in both the assessment of hearing loss and dementia; modifications in a medical regime may successfully eliminate this confounding factor. Using diagnostic therapy, the professional may be able to carefully monitor the efficacy of the intervention approach for signs that more clearly define or reinforce the original diagnosis.

Management

Although dementia is typically considered to be irreversible, it has been documented that hearing loss represents 20–30% of the reversible causes of dementia [65]. Among professionals who work with this population, there have been many anecdotal reports that suggest that in some cases the use of amplification by the client results in improved communication that reflects a higher level of cognitive functioning than has been attributed to an individual. Both these statistics and observations suggest that intervention and use of hearing aids and other hearing assistive technology, as well as aural rehabilitation, may result in the improvement of both communicative and cognitive functioning for the older adult.

7.7 The Biological, Psychological, and Social Effects of Hearing Loss on Older Adults

"Hearing loss has a significant impact on communication abilities and social interactions of older adults" [66]. The inability to communicate effectively because of hearing loss has far reaching effects on older adults and their families. The literature provides ample evidence of these effects on this population biologically, affectively, behaviorally, and cognitively as well as the ability to function in both micro and meso social systems. These factors and many external influences, including societal and cultural views (morays), available health care, related human services, pertaining laws, economic factors, and environmental variables, all affect successful adaptation to hearing loss by older adults. The complex interplay of the biological, psychological, and social effects of hearing loss and these influencing factors have been shown to have a significant influence on overall quality of life for older adults, their families, and friends [67, 68].

7.7.1 Biological Influences

The primary biological characteristics of hearing loss, and which have the greatest bearing on the ability to communicate successfully, are the degree and nature of the loss, age of onset, whether it is progressive, and the rate of progression [69, 70]. Increased stress has also been shown to result from the difficulties associated with hearing loss or where hearing loss is a compounding factor to other disabilities and health conditions. Changes in mobility may also affect the adaptation process [70, 71].

7.7.2 Psychological and Social Contexts

The context of the family and support system is important for understanding adaptation to hearing loss. Family issues include changes in the family through death or divorce, change in family functioning because of illness or disability of a family member, retirement of a spouse (or self), change in economic circumstances, relocation of the family or individual family members, and family perspectives about hearing loss [72–75].

7.7.3 Meso Influences

Hearing loss affects the meso systems in which older adults function including families, work settings, and social contexts. The spouse and other family members are affected in significant ways [74, 76]. Beck, a clinical social worker with a severe hearing loss, identified feelings of helplessness, frustration, and hopelessness in families. Pray [74] identified "parallel reactions" that include failed communication situations experienced by the person with hearing loss and those with whom they communicate. Responses such as frustration, guilt, anxiety, anger, and feelings of incompetence have all been reported in response to the same communication breakdown. Studies by Newman and Weinstein [77] and Quinn [78] document that although spouses are affected by the effects of hearing loss, it is to a lesser extent than the person with hearing loss.

7.7.4 Psychological Influences

The psychological impact of the inability to communicate effectively with family, friends, as well as to achieve normal life functions, may be profound but varies depending on the meaning of the loss to the older individual. This is influenced by personal factors that come into play. Such characteristics may include the capacity of the individual to cope with stress [79], personality [80, 81], adaptability [82], self-concept [83], realistic expectations [84], perspectives on hearing loss [85, 86], motivation [69], and technophobia [81, 87, 88]. Hooker and Shifren [80] provide evidence that certain health conditions may have effects on personality (e.g., multiple sclerosis, stroke). Issues of personality and aging are also addressed by many [81,89,90]. Spirituality and religion are areas that research has consistently shown to be important in people's lives and how they cope with stress and disability [91–93].

Hearing loss, like any other personal loss, may result in grieving processes described by Kubler-Ross [94] including denial, bargaining, anger, and acceptance. Pray [74] questions whether acceptance is an appropriate end process for those with hearing loss and suggests that adaptation may be more critical in situations where change is possible.

Depression and other psychological conditions have been shown to be associated with hearing loss among older individuals [71, 95–97]. Cacciatore et al. [71] noted a strong association between hearing loss and depression, and Bazargan et al. [98] cite studies that document a significant reduction of psychotic activity and improvement in mood, self-sufficiency in instrumental activities of daily living, and social relationships after the fitting of hearing aids [99–101].

Bazargan and Barbe [102] found that older individuals with hearing loss self-reported memory problems. A number of studies have identified reduced cognitive capacity in older adults with hearing loss [71, 103]. The ability to cope may be compounded by lack of information and misinformation available to consumers in various mediums. This periodically occurs in websites from health professionals including doctors (e.g., "There is nothing that can be done about nerve deafness") and perpetuated by some advertising related to hearing aid use (i.e., "You can hear a whisper at 20 feet!"). Other studies of the older population demonstrate a significant relationship between hearing impairment and self-sufficiency [95], quality of life and well-being [104, 105], social integration [106], and social isolation [75, 97].

There are also some factors related to adaptation to significant life events that have been thought to compound the effects of hearing loss but are not supported by the literature. The Duke Center for the Study of Aging and Human Development's second longitudinal study [107] reported data on five major life events: participant's retirement, spouse's retirement, widowhood, departure of last child from home, and occurrence of an illness severe enough to require hospitalization. Few effects on social-psychological adaptation were found as a consequence of spouse's retirement, widowhood, and the departure of the last child. Even major medical events were found to have little lasting impact. The most negative effects were related to the participant's retirement, and even those were considered to be relatively minor [107]. It may be that the response to such events is an indicator of how an individual is able to adapt and may only be significant when they happen concurrently with onset or significant decline in hearing ability. Furthermore, coping skills learned during such events may be utilized in coping with subsequent stressors.

Earlier writings reported these events to have negative outcomes such as unhappiness, loss of self-esteem, withdrawal, and general decline [108–111]. Other literature predating the 25-year longitudinal study at the Duke Center suggested that such life events were stressful but resulted in successful readjustment and new growth [82, 112]. Such results are consistent with favorable outcomes associated with crisis and crisis intervention models, which serve to restore communication function or enhance an individual's ability to interact with the environment. Habilitation or rehabilitation may focus on adaptation to communication differences or disorders, enhancement of communication skills, and the use of technology.

7.7.5 Societal Context

Societal attitudes and values provide a cultural context that influence how and how successfully older adults adjust to hearing loss. Butler [108] introduced the term "ageism" to describe stereotyping of persons moving into old age, drawing comparisons with both sexism and racism. Rosow [111] noted the devalued position of older persons in American society. Orr [113] hypothesized that older persons, in ways similar to that of children and youth, are treated with paternalism and are disenfranchised. Wax [114] described the concept of double and multiple jeopardy with regard to older adults who have hearing loss. However, Markides [115] found mixed support in empirical studies for this concept.

Pray [74] explored a body of literature that posits that disability is defined not by the physical condition or "impairment," but instead by the "spoiled identity" resulting from stigma and alienation [116,117]. Watson and Maxwell [118] maintain that social criteria and not physical criteria determine disability and are based on the person's ability to function in the group. Harvey [89] observes that "hearing loss per se need not be a handicapping deficit; rather, this disability may be molded to become such a deficit in the context of the ecology (xii)."

Cultural influences related to communication affect both reactions to hearing loss and coping ability. In some cultures, all disabilities are perceived as reasons for shame or embarrassment, in others as a spiritual punishment of challenge [119]. Antithetically, there are some cultures who revere those who are "special." Successful coping may require assertive approaches, inappropriate in some cultures, especially for women. In other cultures, direct eye contact with a family patriarch or even a male family member is unacceptable; consider the consequences for speech reading training. The cultural context in which an older adult with hearing loss functions must be regarded carefully by professionals.

7.7.6 External Influences

There are external factors that bear significantly on the ability of older adults to successfully adapt to hearing loss. Among these are health care, economics, law and policy issues, as well as the physical environments in which they communicate.

The type of health care and the extent to which it is available may be problematic to older adults. There is a documented scarcity of broad aural rehabilitation services, including training in communication strategies and providing support for coping with psychosocial issues specifically related to hearing loss [120–122].

Furthermore, access to hearing health care is limited by the types and availability of health insurance held by older adults.

The economic status of older adults also impinges in successful adaptation to hearing loss. Given the limited and fixed incomes of many seniors, many cannot afford comprehensive health insurance. Medicare, however, does provide reimbursement for hearing testing. Unfortunately, the current cost of digital hearing aids often runs in the several thousand dollar range and is not covered by the vast majority of health insurance programs. This puts amplification beyond the reach of many seniors who need them. Interestingly, cochlear implants are covered by health insurance, but this is an appropriate intervention for a very small portion of the older adult population; approximately 22,000 adults are cochlear implant recipients, and fewer of these recipients are over the age of 65 years [123].

Many seniors have little knowledge about hearing loss and the options that may be available to them for coping with this loss. Their general practitioners and internists, likewise, do not always know about the broad range of options currently available. Referrals may be inappropriate or may not be made based on outmoded practice trends that posit that "nerve deafness" is not treatable. Furthermore, dissemination of related information has not kept pace with the technological advancements. By far, the most available information is through commercial sources and is typically biased, focusing primarily on sales of their specific products rather than general hearing health care.

The landmark Americans with Disabilities Act (1992) has had a significant impact on all individuals who are deaf and hard of hearing by protecting their right to access in employment, public services, and other public entities. Reasonable accommodations are required for this population. Again, information about the law and how to get it enforced has not reached the general population.

A final challenge to older Americans is in coping with the physical environments within which they communicate (e.g., home, work, avocational, spiritual). Four environmental factors—acoustic, visual, spatial relationships, and comfort level, may negatively impact communication for older adults with hearing loss. Seniors may not have the knowledge or wherewithal to select the best environments, or initiate changes in environments that are more conducive of good communication.

Broader aural rehabilitative services, when available, can make a dramatic difference in helping older adults with hearing loss cope with the issues discussed here.

7.8 Assessment Issues and Approaches

7.8.1 Clinical Audiological Assessment of Older Adults

The following is an overview of the key components of clinical audiological assessment of older adults. It is important to note that hearing assessment in an older population entails a test battery approach that should be both comprehensive and functionally oriented [90].

7.8.1.1 Case History

Perhaps one of the most important aspects of the audiologic assessment is obtaining a comprehensive case history. Information is gathered regarding an older adult's current and prior otologic and audiologic history. This includes family history of hearing loss, ear surgery, noise exposure, head injury, onset and duration of hearing loss, whether the loss is progressive or fluctuating, presence of tinnitus, dizziness, to name a few areas of inquiry. In addition to a complete medical history, including medications, the case history assesses functional communication abilities and identifies areas of concern to the older adult in their daily life.

7.8.1.2 Otoscopic Evaluation

This component is important for the identification of outer and middle ear disorders that may warrant medical intervention. It is also critical to detect the presence of both collapsed canals and impacted cerumen, both of which have a high prevalence rate in the older population, and impact assessment as well as the use of hearing technology. Diabetic and immunocompromised older adults present special challenges and require extreme caution in management of these issues.

7.8.1.3 Pure Tone Testing

Audiologic testing using pure tones yields information on the degree, nature, and configuration of hearing loss. With an older population, there are certain modifications that need to be considered to allow for both accurate test results and to meet their special needs. In general, it is important to explain all procedures before testing, offering instructions slowly, clearly, and with visual and contextual clues. Verification of understanding, including demonstrating the procedure, is often quite helpful. Modification of the procedures for pure tone testing often includes the use of pulsed tones and longer tonal presentations, along with flexibility in manner of response.

7.8.1.4 Speech Testing

The purpose of this component of the testing is to obtain a profile of an older adult's communicative function by evaluating their speech recognition ability. Typically, the protocol for speech testing with older adults involves a series of tests. These tests are conducted to determine performance under a variety of presentation levels, conditions (e.g., quiet and in the presence of background noise), and by comparing speech understanding by listening alone, or in combination with vision and contextual information. This, in turn, provides information that is helpful to determine an older adult's potential benefit from amplification and other hearing assistive technologies.

7.8.1.5 Immittance Testing

Acoustic immittance measures are used with older adults to evaluate the status of the middle ear system. The test battery includes tympanometry and acoustic stapedial reflex testing. Research in this area has shown that norms for adults can be applied to older adults.

7.8.1.6 Electrophysiological Measures

Testing using auditory brainstem response (ABR) assesses neural transmission through the central nervous system, which may change as part of the aging process. ABR testing in older adults is affected by many variables including, but not limited to, body temperature, collapsed canals, hearing loss, and muscular artifacts. In addition to establishing separate norms for older adults on this measure, specific assessment protocols for auditory potentials in older adults have been recommended. Another component of electrophysiologic testing is otoacoustic emissions testing (OAE). This test provides information about the function of the cochlea, and outer hair cell function in particular.

7.8.2 Consideration of Test Adaptations and Modifications with Older Adults

Slower response time—modifications may include slowing down tonal presentation and allowing the older adult to set the pace for interstimulus intervals.
Failing attention because of medications/illness—consider keeping the sessions short, no longer than 45–60 min, with breaks if fatigue starts to set in.
Movement deficits—modifications to consider include trying different strategies for responses before the start of testing; use a response strategy that is most natural and reflexive.
Memory deficits—repeat and simplify instructions, adding gestures to supplement instructions and allow lots of practice, frequent reconditioning, and positive reinforcement.

7.8.3 Communication and Psychosocial Needs Assessment for Intervention

7.8.3.1 Self-Assessment Scales of Communication Function

The Communication Self-Assessment Scales for Older Adults (CSOA), developed by Kaplan et al. [124], comprises a 41-item Communication Strategies scale and includes another important scale, a 31-item Communication Attitudes scale. Standardized on a population of 135 independent-living adults with hearing loss, ranging in age from 60 to 88 years, it can be used to evaluate the communication strategies and attitudes of an individual older adult client. Results provide a basis for designing aural rehabilitation intervention. In addition, the scale can be used to show changes in the use of communication strategies and attitudes of a group of clients 3 and 9 months after completion of aural rehabilitation programs.

Another self-assessment scale that is often used with older adults is the Hearing Handicap Inventory for the Elderly (HHIE), developed by Ventry and Weinstein [75]. This scale was standardized on noninstitutionalized older adults. Comprising 25 items, its content focuses on areas of social and emotional function.

For older adults residing in a nursing home environment, Schow and Nerbonne [125] introduced the Nursing Home Hearing Handicap Scale. A separate version of the scale can be given to staff members and/or family members to indicate areas of communication difficulty that they perceive to be a problem, which may corroborate or differ from the older adult's self-assessed difficulty resulting from their hearing loss. This in turn can help direct counseling with the older adult. As with the above-mentioned scales, the Nursing Home Hearing Handicap Scale can also be used as a measure to evaluate effectiveness of intervention and rehabilitation.

7.8.3.2 Receptive Communication Needs Assessment for Hearing Assistive Technology

As a hearing aid and/or cochlear implant user, older adults have firsthand experience with technologies that can help them communicate. However, as described in Section 7.6, even when they use amplification many older adults continue to experience difficulty hearing and understanding in some situations, particularly in noise and at a distance. To help individuals with hearing loss obtain full communication access, the Rehabilitation Engineering Research Center on Hearing Enhancement (RERC) at Gallaudet University [126] has developed a comprehensive questionnaire, the Hearing Assistive Technology Needs Assessment Profile (HATNAP), to systematically identify the unique communication needs of each individual.

The HATNAP is a needs assessment tool that provides specific recommendations for hearing assistance technologies and communication strategies designed to improve an older adult's ability to hear and understand in all situations of their life. The HATNAP also helps determine what training and strategies may be necessary to facilitate meeting the communication needs that were identified by the older adult. The original conception of this assessment tool grew out of extensive work by Compton that began in the 1980s in the area of assistive technology, culminating in the founding of Gallaudet's Assistive Device Center, an earlier version of this questionnaire on assistive technology [127], and efforts to promote the use of assistive technology in the professional community.

Hearing loss or not, all people share the following four receptive communication needs [127, 128]:

1. Face-to-face communication (one-to-one or in groups);
2. Enjoyment of electronic media (radio, stereo system, television, movie sound tracks, among others);

3. Telephone communication (home and office, cellular, pay phone);
4. Awareness of important warning sounds (doorbell, smoke alarm, pager, to name a few).

Because of recent technological advancements, today's hearing aids and cochlear implants do an excellent job of helping older adults meet these needs. However, there are often situations where additional technologies may be needed. For example, older adults may continue to experience difficulty understanding speech in noisy environments or from a distance, such as when dining out, listening to a lecture, or attending a movie or play. Understanding speech over the telephone can be difficult, even in quiet, because no visual cues are present. At bedtime, even those older adults with a mild-to-moderate hearing loss may not hear the smoke alarm located down the hall and behind a closed door if they are in a deep sleep and their hearing aids have been removed for the night. They may also miss a doorbell chime while listening to the TV a room away. These are all issues that impact the safety, security, independence, and well being of an older adult.

In addition to hearing aids and cochlear implants, there is an entire range of hearing assistance technology (HAT) available to help older adults in these situations. Furthermore, this technology can help individuals with all degrees of hearing loss. There is HAT that can help older adults hear better on the phone, at a movie theater, at restaurants, in meetings, while watching TV or listening to music, to name a few. There are even devices that can alert them to when someone is at the door, when the telephone is ringing, or when the smoke alarm is activated. There may even be features already installed in the older adult's hearing aid/implant that can be used not only to enhance listening on the telephone but also to improve understanding in situations such as while watching TV or conversing in a restaurant or meeting. It is this range of technology that can help an older adult have full communication access and facilitate their independence and quality of life overall.

Although hearing assistive technology has been available for over 30 years, there have been limited attempts to systematically determine candidacy and to offer this technology to hearing impaired individuals. Initial work in this area was begun by Vaughn and Lightfoot [129], and Palmer and Garstecki [130]. Recent advances in technology and outcome measures have sparked the development of other assessment tools [131, 132] that promote a continuum of hearing technologies for professionals to consider. Some of the leading work in the area of hearing assistive technology over the last 20 years has been done by Compton [127, 133], providing a model for the development of assistive device centers and serving as a national resource on this technology.

The Hearing Assistance Technology Needs Assessment Profile (HATNAP) developed at Gallaudet University systematically assesses individual receptive communication needs in four key areas: face-to-face communication, reception of media, telephone communication, and awareness of alerting signals. The assessment goes into great depth in each of these areas and covers communication performance in an extensive variety of listening situations at home, at work, during leisure activities for each of the four key assessment areas. For example, in the area of telephone use, the HATNAP first establishes for each location (e.g. home, work, leisure) the type of phone that is primarily used (e.g., cordless phone at home). The next step identifies the strategies that the individual is using. Stated differently, how is the person using the phone at present (e.g., do they hold the phone up to the microphone of their hearing aid and use a telephone amplifier). Once the phone type is identified for each location, along with the strategy of use, then a determination is made of the success or difficulty that the person is having. A 5-point Lickert scale is used to determine a person's experience in a particular listening situation, with a range from "rarely have difficulty" to "always have difficulty." This allows the professional to identify both technology and strategies to resolve areas where the person continues to have problems. This same approach is used with other areas of receptive communication needs. In all, the HATNAP offers a comprehensive need assessment for hearing assistive technology that is not found elsewhere.

What is also unique about the HATNAP is the inclusion of tutorials on hearing assistive technology. This new assessment tool will be placed into an interactive computer format with educational material that can benefit older consumers and professionals alike. A great deal of expertise is often needed to make appropriate recommendations for technology. Research underway is working on the development of a decision tree to be integrated into the computer software for the HATNAP. This decision-making process will take an individual's needs assessment profile and then yield specific solution sets for both technology and strategies.

Problem-solving strategies, training, and counseling with hearing assistive technology are as critical to successful use as the technology itself. Research has shown that older adults in particular have a great deal of difficulty asserting their needs and requesting that others wear a microphone, for example. In no small measure, despite dramatic improvement in signal-to-noise ratio, and better understanding of speech, many older adults are uncomfortable with this aspect of some assistive hearing technology. This, in turn, limits its use and the greater independence and well being that go along with it. Innovative approaches that are discussed in the next section may be key to the acceptance of this technology by an older adult.

7.9 Interventions and Technologies for Independence and Well-Being

7.9.1 Personal Hearing Instruments

7.9.1.1 Hearing Aids

Hearing aids are designed to amplify ambient sounds and deliver the amplified signals to the impaired ear. Because hearing loss results in a loss of sensitivity to soft sounds, gain is provided so that they become loud enough to be heard. However, gain cannot be uniformly applied across all speech frequencies, because hearing loss typically affects different frequency regions differently. Nor should gain be provided in the same way for input signals of all levels, or else many of the sounds of daily life would be made so loud as to be intolerable to the user. As it happens, people with sensory hearing loss, which results from a loss of sensory hair cells in the cochlea, the most common type of hearing loss in older adults, are subject to a phenomenon known as recruitment, which can be briefly described as an abnormal growth of loudness. That is, while softer sounds may be inaudible, louder sounds are perceived to be as loud as they would be without the presence of hearing loss. Thus, hearing aids must control the amount of gain provided for input signals of differing amplitude and frequency.

Hearing Aid Configurations

There are several styles of hearing aids, differing in size, shape, and coupling to the ear. Arranged according to size from larger to smaller, they are body, behind-the-ear (BTE), in-the-ear (ITE), in-the-canal (ITC), and completely-in-the-canal (CIC) hearing aids.

Body hearing aids are the oldest style, rarely found in today's market. Consisting of a body-worn case with a microphone, a cord, a button receiver, and an earmold, this style of hearing aid minimizes acoustic feedback in the case of profound hearing loss where gain is substantial. It also has the virtue of being easier to manipulate, having larger batteries and controls. A BTE hearing aid consists of a head-worn case that houses the microphone and electronics and fits behind the pinna of the external ear, and a tone hook that connects to acoustic tubing, which in turn connects to an earmold. This configuration is most common in people with more severe or profound hearing loss because of their gain requirements and the problem of acoustic feedback. The greater distance (relative to an ITE or ITC style of aid) between the amplified signal and the microphone of the hearing aid helps to reduce the likelihood of feedback. This type of hearing aid has the virtue of being larger, so that those with visual and fine-motor limitations may find it easier to manage. The larger size is also a disadvantage for many users who have cosmetic concerns about the hearing aid's visibility. In contrast, ITE, ITC, and CIC hearing aids are much smaller and fit entirely into the concha (ITE) or ear canal (ITC or CIC), obviating the need for a separate earmold. The case is custom-made to fit snugly and form a seal between the ear canal and the outside air, in order to control feedback. The microphone is typically placed on the face of the hearing aid and thus is placed in a natural position at the entrance of the ear canal. Although these smaller sized hearing aids are valued for their reduced visibility, there is a cost in increased possibility of feedback because of the proximity of the microphone to the amplified signal from the hearing aid.

Digital Hearing Aids

For many years, hearing aids have been essentially miniature amplifiers with electronic circuits designed to amplify, filter, and control the levels of signals. However, since the development of computer chips that are very small, powerful, efficient, and able to operate at low power, digital hearing aids have become the industry standard. Such aids contain computer circuits that convert sound into numerical representations that can be transformed mathematically and converted back into sound for delivery to the ear. Digital hearing aids provide for greater flexibility and adaptability in fitting, permitting more precise frequency shaping, as well as the implementation of complex signal-processing algorithms. They also allow hearing aids to have multiple memories, so that users can select among two or more different fittings that have been specially tuned for specific environments such as noisy restaurants, telephone calls, children's voices, and others. A problem with digital hearing aids is their complexity. It is a challenge for an audiologist to achieve the "best fit" for hearing aids in which a large number of variables are at play. For this reason, digital hearing aids are typically marketed with software that implements fitting strategies unique to the features of the particular hearing aid. Audiologists are faced with the challenge of having multiple software applications, often from different hearing aid companies. Thankfully, there is a standard computer interface that was developed by a consortium of hearing aid companies that permits audiologists to work with multiple brands using the same hardware interface, known as NOAH.

Frequency Selectivity

As mentioned earlier, hearing loss affects different frequency regions of hearing differently. Typically, hearing in the higher frequency regions tends to be more greatly affected than lower frequency regions for older adults, although this is not always the case. At first blush, it may seem logical to provide gain that is equivalent to the hearing loss and therefore to "mirror" the hearing loss with amplification. In practice, however, this is not desirable because of recruitment. Much hearing aid research in the early years of electronic hearing aids was focused on how much gain to provide at each frequency for maximum speech perception performance and comfort (an excellent review is provided in Dillon [134]). Various prescriptive formulae have been worked out, and over time, the formulae have become more complex as hearing aid technology has become more sophisticated. Digital hearing aids are fit by Audiologists using software in which one or more prescriptive formulae have been implemented. In some cases, these formulae are based on hearing thresholds and in others on loudness judgments.

Control of Loudness

Because of recruitment, a common phenomenon affecting older adults with hearing loss, loudness must be controlled in hearing aids to prevent discomfort and possible additional damage to hearing, as well as to maximize speech intelligibility. Hearing aids often use amplitude compression, also known as automatic gain control (AGC) or automatic volume control (AVC), to adjust the growth of loudness and limit output. Simple AGC circuits control gain across all frequencies simultaneously, but because an individual's hearing loss, and therefore recruitment, may be different in different frequency regions, multi-channel hearing aids have been developed in which different AGC characteristics are applied to two or three separate bands of frequency. Adaptive compression circuits have been used in advanced hearing aids.

Such circuits are designed to modify their temporal parameters (attack time, release time) depending on the characteristics of the incoming sound. Thus, sounds with rapid changes in amplitude, such as impulsive sounds, are treated differently by the circuit than sounds that change their amplitude more slowly, resulting in improved user comfort.

Noise Reduction

Consumers' most common complaints about their hearing aids involve their performance in backgrounds of noise [135]. Many attempts at reducing the effects of noise have been made, but single-microphone noise reduction in hearing aids has been largely unsuccessful in improving speech understanding in noise [136]. Currently, there is a great deal of interest in directional-microphone hearing aids, which are most sensitive to sounds coming from the front and suppress sounds from the rear and sides. Their design is based on the assumption that users will want to hear best in the direction in which they are looking, and that noise sources will be more likely to arise from other directions. This may not always be the case, because listening situations can vary greatly. In some situations, users may prefer to have an omni-directional pattern so that they can monitor the environment in all directions; in other situations, users may prefer a highly directional pattern in order to improve the signal-to-noise ratio of the desired speech. Current hearing aids are often equipped with switches that permit the user to choose a directional pattern that suits the situation.

7.9.1.2 Cochlear Implants

In the case of people with hearing loss so severe that hearing aids provide only limited or no benefit, cochlear implants are now an option. Although hearing aids amplify and deliver sound to an impaired inner ear, cochlear implants bypass the cochlea and directly stimulate the neurons of the auditory system with electrical pulses that result in auditory sensations. A cochlear implant system consists of both external and internal components. Externally worn components include a microphone, a speech processor, and a head-worn transmitter; internal components include a receiver/stimulator that is placed behind the ear and fixed to the skull and a connected electrode array that is threaded into one of the ducts (the scala tympani) of the cochlea. Naturally, a surgical procedure is required to put the internal components in place. This usually takes place on an out-patient basis, and after a period of healing of about 1 month, the external components are fit and the stimulation is turned on. Although early cochlear implants consisted of head-worn microphones and body-worn speech processors, contemporary cochlear implants have very small processors that are worn behind the ear, like hearing aids. Sound is picked up by the microphone, which is typically mounted at the ear, similar to a BTE hearing aid. The sound is then processed by the speech processor, and the processed signal is transmitted across the skin to the internal receiver through a head-worn transmitter. The internal receiver accepts the signal from the transmitter and performs the final operation: that of sending trains of electrical pulses to the assigned electrodes in the array. The array consists of a number of electrodes arranged tonotopically along the cochlea, that is to say representing frequencies from low (at the end of the array, deepest into the cochlea) to high (toward the entry point of the array).

Although stimulation is typically turned on about 1 month post implant surgery, it can take many months or years for an individual to gain full benefit from a cochlear implant; there is also much variability in patient outcomes. Some people appear to receive immediate and substantial benefits, such as being able to talk on the telephone, whereas others receive only limited benefit even after many years. There are many factors that are related to outcomes with cochlear implants, including age at onset of deafness, duration of deafness before implantation, number of surviving neurons in the cochlea, and many others, some of which are not well understood. Candidacy for a cochlear implant is largely determined by these considerations as well as the level of residual hearing [137]. The Food and Drug Administration [FDA] has established candidacy guidelines for adults and children for each of the approved devices. Whereas in prior years, surgery was often not recommended with older adults, older adults are now considered candidates for cochlear implants and have demonstrated successful outcomes. Cochlear implants have been found to have a significant impact on the quality of life of older adults with profound hearing loss [138].

Cochlear implant stimulation is limited in its ability to reproduce sound sensations, and even those who may perform well in terms of speech understanding may have great difficulty appreciating music [139]. One reason for this is the fact that unlike natural hearing, cochlear implant stimulation is an extracted coded signal that is generated by the speech processor of the implant. The function of the speech processor is to convert the audio signal into a set of instructions for stimulating the electrodes in the array. The instructions vary according to the speech-processing strategy that is chosen and the individual's sensitivity to electrical stimulation. When fitting the cochlear implant, an audiologist measures the user's sensitivity by conducting a behavioral evaluation of thresholds for just-detectable and most comfortable levels of electrical stimulation for each electrode in the array. The patient's threshold and comfort levels are stored in the speech processor and used in the process of encoding sound into electrical stimulation of the electrode array.

In representing speech, it is important to provide detailed spectral and temporal information. The speech processor provides spectral information to the user by filtering the signal into several frequency bands, extracting the envelope of the signal in each band, and using it to modulate a series of electrical pulses that are delivered to a corresponding electrode along the array. Temporal information is provided through rapid sampling of the signal and updating of the stimulation at the electrodes. The relative value to speech understanding of these two parameters in cochlear implants is not fully understood. Different speech-processing strategies emphasize temporal and spectral information to differing degrees. Each of the strategies now being used has been successful in helping many users understand speech, although adults who are fit with cochlear implants appear to be quite definite about which strategy they prefer [140]. There are several different speech-processing strategies, and they differ in their availability according to the implant manufacturer. Each implant offers two or more options from which the user, guided by the audiologist, chooses one that sounds most acceptable and yields the best speech understanding. Upon initial stimulation, more than one option is made available because the speech processors contain two or more memories in which different strategies may be stored.

7.9.2 Hearing Assistive Technology

People with hearing loss have an increased susceptibility to the effects of noise and distance [141, 142], and speech perception performance of people using cochlear implants deteriorates substantially with background noise [143]. For this reason, hearing assistive technologies [also referred to as assistive listening systems (ALS) or assistive listening devices (ALD)] have been developed to help manage problems caused by reverberation and ambient noise found in many environments such as theaters, places of worship, schools, auditoriums, and arenas. The basic principle is simple: a microphone is placed close to the desired sound source (e.g., on the speaker's lapel) and coupled to an individual's ear (as when using a headphone), hearing aid, or cochlear implant. Although hard-wire connections may still be used in some situations, generally ALDS use three different wireless media to transmit and receive signals: magnetic induction (induction loops or IL), frequency-modulated radio frequencies (FM) and infrared (IR) light.

7.9.2.1 Hard-Wire Systems

The simplest and least expensive assistive listening system available is a hard-wired personal amplifier, which consists of a microphone, an amplifier, and a transducer. An example of such a system is the Pocketalker, produced by Williams Sound (www.williamssound.com). The virtue of such systems are their simplicity and low cost. They can serve as general-use amplifiers for situations in which hearing aids are not available. They also serve as ALS when the microphone is placed in proximity to the sound source and connected by a wire to the amplifier and the listener. This can be particularly useful in noisy restaurants or other noisy conditions, as well as in emergency situations. An example of the latter is that of a person with a hearing loss in a hospital without his or her hearing aids. A Pocketalker may be used as a temporary measure to help facilitate communication with caregivers and physicians. Such systems have an additional advantage when confidentiality is important, such as in counseling situations. Whereas wireless systems broadcast information so that it could possibly be picked up by others, a hard-wire system is completely private.

7.9.2.2 Magnetic Induction

The first application of magnetic induction to assistive hearing was intended to facilitate telephone listening. Early telephone handsets created magnetic fields around the earpiece as an unintended byproduct. Telecoils in hearing aids were designed to pick up the modulations of the magnetic field and present the signal to the user. Telephones that work in this way with hearing aids are said to be hearing aid compatible. Both wire line and wireless telephones manufactured for sale in the USA are required to be hearing aid compatible.

For those hearing aids equipped with telecoils, the telecoil functions not only to assist with improved understanding on phones but in a broader way as a means to interface with assistive hearing technology systems. Magnetic induction has been widely applied in group listening systems. In such so-called loop systems, a loop of wire is placed around a room (floor or ceiling height). The desired signal (from a microphone or other sound system) is amplified and passed through the loop, setting up a modulated magnetic field. Hearing aid wearers switch their hearing aids to telecoil mode (T) or telecoil/microphone (TM) mode to hear the signal. For users who do not have hearing aids with telecoils, magnetic induction receivers are available that can be used with headphones.

Magnetic induction can also serve as an interface between other assistive technologies and a hearing aid or cochlear implant that has a telecoil. A neck loop or silhouette can be used for this purpose. A neck loop is a kind of miniature teleloop system; a loop of wire is worn around the neck connected by a plug (typically 3.5-mm mini phone plug) to any audio device that has a compatible socket, such as an MP3 player, radio, television, or FM/IR assistive device. A silhouette is similar in function, although it substitutes the loop of wire with a thin wafer, shaped like a BTE hearing aid that sits on the ear in proximity to the hearing aid. A wire connects the silhouette to any input device with a compatible socket.

A significant advantage of magnetic induction is that no receiver is needed for a user with a hearing aid or cochlear implant equipped with a telecoil. It solves many listening problems of hearing aid or cochlear implant wearers, and can be found on most telephones. Unfortunately, not all hearing aids in the USA are dispensed with a telecoil, which limits the usefulness of teleloop systems. Magnetic induction systems do not provide privacy, and the signals have a tendency to spillover to adjacent rooms. Interference is an additional problem that sometimes arises to bedevil hearing aid users. Sources include some kinds of lighting, cathode ray tubes, backlit displays on telephones, and other electrical appliances and devices. Unfortunately, the only solution available when confronted with magnetic interference is to identify and turn off the source of the interference, or move to another location.

7.9.2.3 FM Systems

FM systems act as miniature independent radio transmitters, broadcasting the desired signal to the audience. The signals may be live speech or music picked up by a microphone, or other signals such as soundtracks, that are connected through line input to the FM transmitter from an existing public address system. The user must have a receiver that is tuned to the same frequency channel as the transmitter. FM systems use the same radio signal as commercial FM radio, but they use specific frequency bands (72–75 MHz and 216–217 MHz) that are essentially unregulated and used for personal radio in the USA (Code of Federal Regulations, 47CFR2.106). The maximum permissible power of an assistive listening system is 80 mV/m at 3 m, which can be effective between 300 and 500 feet. Somewhat greater operating distances are possible with the 216–217 MHz band. Such devices are low in power and not likely to interfere with other permitted users in the same channels (i.e., paging devices, emergency vehicles). No priority is given to ALD; in the event of interference, a user must switch to another channel within the same frequency band.

An advantage of FM is the fact that the coverage is fairly uniform over the effective range. Although interference from other sources of radio energy is possible, such problems are not common and can be dealt with by changing the frequency of transmission. A disadvantage of FM transmission is the ease with which it can be received makes public performances more susceptible to pirating. There have been reports of performers not agreeing to use FM systems for this reason. For the same reasons, when private information is being exchanged FM is not the technology of choice.

7.9.2.4 IR Systems

IR systems use light outside the visible spectrum (∼700–1000 nm) as a medium for transmission. Channels are band-limited to reduce interference from other sources of light and heat. The light carrier is modulated by a sub-carrier frequency, usually 95 kHz, although this can vary among systems. A transmitter encodes the desired audio signal and sends it to the emitter (an array of light-emitting diodes), which beams the light to the receivers in the audience. An IR receiver always has a lens and a photo-detecting diode that is capable of picking up the IR light signal. An optical filter on the lens helps reduce interference. The receiver demodulates the sub-carrier, and the audio signal is retrieved and amplified for listening. Direct line of sight is usually required for IR to work effectively (as in a television remote control). Bright sunlight will interfere with the signal and add static, although some systems are quite successful in reducing light interference.

In situations where privacy is important, IR offers a good choice because the transmission can be contained within the room, unlike FM or magnetic induction systems in which there is considerable spill-over of the signal into surrounding areas. This makes IR particularly appealing to the entertainment industry.

7.10 Special Considerations in the Selection and Use of Technologies for Older Adults

Lesner [144] offers an excellent review of the myriad of candidacy and management issues associated with the use of hearing aid technology and older adults. Ideally, the identification of an older adult's comprehensive communication needs and their need for hearing assistive technology should be an integral part of the initial diagnostic and rehabilitation planning. An older adult's continuum of communication needs may best be served with assistive technology, either alone or in combination with amplification. Approaching this from a total rehabilitation framework enables the best selection of hearing technology, and maximizes the success of audiologic intervention with the ultimate goal of helping the older adult attain independence and better quality of life afforded by improved communication.

In addition to aspects of audiologic status that enter into decisions about amplification and assistive technology, some of the salient coexisting candidacy issues that affect older adults include, but are not limited to, biologic/physical concerns such as visual impairment and dexterity difficulties [66, 145]. Arthritis, one of the most common chronic conditions facing older adults [146], often presents the older adult with pain and can compromise dexterity, both of which can limit the use of hearing aids by older adults [147]. The provision of assistive technology that is both larger and simpler to control can offer the older adult with dexterity and/or visual problems a means to overcome these difficulties and facilitate successful use of technology. According to Lesner [144] "perhaps the most important factor when considering ALDs for older adults is the simplicity of operation." For older adults with cognitive impairment, hearing assistive technology can also be a very useful alternative to hearing aids because they are simpler to use. This, in turn, can yield a degree of independence that would otherwise be unavailable, with improved day-to-day function for everyday communication, a critical component of both stimulation and connection to their environment.

Psychosocial factors, especially depression, can also have a bearing on the use of hearing technology. Some claim that use may be limited by the loss of motivation to communicate [148]. However, it may be that the lack of auditory stimulation itself contributes to isolation and depression. Because the primary impact of hearing loss is on the ability to communicate with others, providing hearing technology can have a significant effect on the day-to-day life of an older adult, affecting their participation in activities of daily life and improving their overall well being.

Environmental factors including listening in noise, at a distance, and in a reverberant condition have been shown to be very difficult situations for older adults, and impact a range of lifestyles from those who are bed-ridden to those who are very active. HAT, either used separately or with amplification (e.g., FM system incorporated into a personal hearing aid) is able to overcome many of these difficulties, providing a significant improvement in the signal-to-noise ratio, thereby making the speaker's voice easier to hear and improving communication overall. Although assistive technology can offer a viable alternative or addition to traditional hearing aids, there are issues related to the acceptance and use of this technology that need to be considered as well. In addition to professional involvement, Lesner [144] and Riemer-Reiss and Wacker [149] stress the importance of patient involvement in the selection process as a key factor in ensuring its success. This runs counter to the medical model where decisions are made for the individual.

7.11 Aural Rehabilitation

Defining aural rehabilitation, Mark Ross [150] states that "it includes, in my judgment, any device, procedure, information, interaction, or therapy which lessens the communicative and psychosocial consequences of a hearing loss."

Structured, formal AR programs have been consistently shown to be effective and beneficial for people with hearing loss, improving audio-visual speech recognition performance, psychosocial functioning, and reducing hearing aid returns [151–156].

Unfortunately, few audiologists provide comprehensive aural rehabilitation services. Research has shown that the hearing needs of hard of hearing and deaf people are addressed most often by the provision of technological aids such as hearing aids and cochlear implants. Fitting of ALD is often conducted in an informal way. Provision of other services that would lead to better communicative competence is rarely carried out in formal programs.

A survey of audiologists conducted in 1990 indicated that only 23% were providing communication training such as speech reading and auditory training: a decrease from 38% in 1980 [120]. Carmen [121] recently described the results of an online survey of audiologists. Of 217 respondents, 85% reported dispensing hearing aids, but only 24% reported that they provided "aural rehabilitation classes." Sixty-five percent reported that they did provide "therapeutic counseling," which was defined as "helping patients overcome the emotional influences caused by hearing loss." Another recent survey of audiologists (110 respondents) about the frequency of provision of AR services [122] revealed that although audiologists frequently provide information about ALD (84%), communication strategies training (83%), and informational counseling (82%), they less frequently provided information about coping strategies (57%), psychosocial adjustment (45%), and partner training (38%). The most neglected areas of aural rehabilitation were auditory training (~18% provided services) and speechreading (only ~6% provided services).

This dearth of comprehensive aural rehabilitation services is further compounded by external factors that influence older adults such as economics, culture, health care scope and availability, insurance coverage, transportation, accessibility, legislation, and the effects of societal stigma. Faced with the complexity of issues both within the field of audiology to provide adequate rehabilitation services, coupled with issues that confront older adults overall, and the burgeoning numbers of baby boomers, it compels us to come up with new service models and approaches to meet the needs of older adults with hearing loss.

Several such programs are currently under evaluation, including the Gallaudet University Peer Mentoring Training Program and the American Academy of Hearing Loss Support Specialists of the Hearing Loss Association of America (HLAA). The Gallaudet Program is designed for individuals with hearing loss who have successfully adjusted and wish to provide support to other person with hearing loss. Students complete a 2-year nonresidential graduate degree certificate program, modeled after mentor training programs designed for other health care professions. It includes both academic and experiential learning. In contrast, the HLAA program is designed to help anyone with an interest in hearing loss to learn more about it in a four-course academic online program with the objective of providing support to individuals with hearing loss. The programs were designed collaboratively and both address significant areas including technology orientation, nature of hearing loss, interpretation of test results, resources and services, expectations and outcomes, environmental modifications, and psychosocial adaptation. Environmental modification focuses on creating and restructuring better communication contexts. Psychosocial adaptation may include emotional support, behavior modification, cognitive restructuring, normalization and validation, assertiveness training, as well as the effective use of communication strategies.

Greater emphasis is now being given to group aural rehabilitation experiences that have proven effective in multiple studies as summarized by Hawkins [157]. In addition, online and computer-based programs are also emerging, making use of the latest technology. Sweetow and Henderson-Sabes [158] offer a self-directed home-based interactive listening and communication training program for adults with hearing loss.

7.12 Summary and Conclusions

This chapter has provided an overview of hearing loss and aging. The authors have described the changing demographics of older adults and the unique ways in which hearing loss affects their lives from biological, psychological, and social perspectives. The impact of several external influences on this population has also been described. Of primary importance is the response of professionals who work with this population in developing and refining assessment approaches for, and selection of, hearing assistive technology. Emphasis has also been placed on creating assessment tools and innovative therapy approaches that address the communication needs and limitations of older adults and ensure more successful adaptation to new technologies. Enhanced communicative functioning through a combination of assistive technology and psychological adjustment contributes to the enhancement of both the independence and quality of life for older adults. Such collaborative and interdisciplinary approaches may provide the strongest foundation for addressing the challenges of hearing loss in aging.

References

1. Kochkin S. MarkeTrak VII: Hearing loss population top 31 million people. *Hear Rev* 2005; 12(7):16–29.
2. Lethbridge-Cejku M, Schiller JS, Bernadel L. Summary health statistics for U.S. adults: National Health Interview Survey. Vital and Health Statistics, 10 (222):1–151. Hyattsville, MD: National Center for Health Statistics, 2004.
3. National Center for Health Statistics. Provisional Report: Summary Health Statistics for U.S. Adults. National Health Interview Survey, 2004. Series 10, Number 228. Hyattsville, MD: National Center for Health Statistics, 2005.

4. Steinmetz E. Americans with Disabilities: 2002, Current Population Reports, P70-170. Washington, DC: U.S. Census Bureau, 2006.
5. Centers for Disease Control and Prevention. Vital and health statistics trends in the health of older Americans: United States, 1994. Washington, DC: US Department of Health and Human Services, 1995.
6. Brock D, Guralnick J, Brody J. Demography and epidemiology of aging in the United States. In: Schneider E, Rose J, eds. *Handbook of the Biology of Aging*, 3rd ed. San Diego: Academic Press, 1990:3–23.
7. National Center for Health Statistics. Aging in the eighties: functional limitations of individuals 65 years and over. Advance data from vital health statistics. No. 133, Hyattsville, MD: Public Health Service, 1987. (DHHS publication no. (PHS) 87–1250.)
8. Garahan MB, Waller JA, Houghton M, Tisdale WA, Runge CF. Hearing loss prevalence and management in nursing home residents. *J Am Geriatr Soc* 1992; 40(2):130–134.
9. Schow R, Nerbonne M, eds. *Introduction to Audiologic Rehabilitation*, 4th ed. Boston, MA: Allyn and Bacon, 2002.
10. Voeks S, Gallagher C, Langer E, Drinka P. Hearing loss in the nursing home: an institutional issue. *J Am Geriatr Soc* 1990; 38:141–145.
11. Abrams W, Beers M, Berkow R. *Merck Manual of Geriatrics*, 2nd ed. Whitehouse Station, NJ: Merck & Co., Inc., 1995.
12. Goodman A. Reference zero levels for pure-tone audiometer. *ASHA* 1965; 7: 262–263.
13. Clark JG. Uses and abuses of hearing loss classification. *ASHA* 1981; 23(7):493–500.
14. Gates GA, Cooper JC, Kannel WB, Miller NJ. Hearing in the elderly: the Framingham cohort, 1983-1985. Part I. Basic audiometric test results. *Ear Hear* 1990; 11(4):247–256.
15. Pearson JD, Morrell CH, Gordon-Salant S, Brant LJ, Metter EJ, Klein LL, et al. Gender differences in a longitudinal study of age-associated hearing loss. *J Acoust Soc Am* 1995; 97(2):1196–1205.
16. American Tinnitus Association. About Tinnitus (Accessed January 6, 2007, at http:www.ata.org/about_tinnitus/).
17. Adams PF, Hendershot GE, Marano MA. Current Estimates from the National Health Interview Survey, 1996. Vital and Health Statistics, 10 (200) (Accessed January 8, 2007, at http://www.cdc.gov/nchs/data/series/sr_10/sr10_200.pdf).
18. United States Department of Commerce. Profiles of General Demographic Characteristics, Washington, DC: U.S. Census Bureau, 2001 (Accessed January 6, 2007, at http://www.census.gov/prod/cen2000/dp1/2kh00.pdf).
19. Henry JA, Dennis KC, Schechter MA. General review of tinnitus: prevalence, mechanisms, effects, and management. *J Speech Lang Hear Res* 2005; 48(5):1204–1235.
20. Luxon LM. Tinnitus: its causes, diagnosis, and treatment. *BMJ* 1993; 306:1490–1491.
21. Perry BP, Gantz BJ. Medical and surgical evaluation and management of tinnitus. In: Tyler RS, ed. *Tinnitus Handbook*. San Diego, CA: Singular, 2000:221–241.
22. Meikle MB, Creedon TA, Griest SE. *Tinnitus Archive*, 2nd ed, 2004. (Accessed January 8, 2007, at http://www.tinnitusArchive.org/).
23. Tyler R. *Tinnitus Handbook*. San Diego, CA: Singular Publishing Group, 2000.
24. Cutson TM. Falls in the elderly. *Am Fam Physician* 1994; 49(1):149–156.
25. Kippenbrock T, Soja ME. Preventing falls in the elderly: interviewing patients who have fallen. Researchers attempt to identify fall-risk factors from the patients' point of view. *Geriatr Nurs* 1993;14(4):205–209.
26. Moscicki EK, Elkins EF, Baum HM, McNamara PM. Hearing loss in the elderly: an epidemiologic study of the Framingham Heart Study Cohort. *Ear Hear* 1985; 6(4):184–190.
27. Cooper JC. Health and Nutrition Examination Survey of 1971–75: Part I. Ear and race effects in hearing. *J Am Acad Audiol* 1994; 5(1):30–36.
28. Gates GA, Cooper JC. Incidence of hearing decline in the elderly. *Acta Otolaryngol* 1991; 111(2):240–248.

29. Brant LJ, Gordon-Salant S, Pearson JD, Klein LL, Morrell CH, Metter EJ, et al. Risk factors related to age-associated hearing loss in the speech frequencies. *J Am Acad Audiol* 1996; 7(3):152–160.
30. Cruickshanks KJ, Wiley TL, Tweed TS, Klein BE, Klein R, Mares-Perlman JA, et al. Prevalence of hearing loss in older adults in Beaver Dam, Wisconsin. The Epidemiology of Hearing Loss Study. *Am J Epidemiol* 1998; 148(9):879–886.
31. Schuknecht HF, Gacek MR. Cochlear pathology in presbycusis. *Ann Otol Rhinol Laryngol* 1993; 102:1–16.
32. Henderson D, Bielefeld EC, Harris KC, Hu BH. The role of oxidative stress in noise-induced hearing loss. *Ear Hear* 2006; 27(1):1–9.
33. Campbell KC, Rybak LP, Meech RP, Hughes L. D-methionine provides excellent protection from cisplatin ototoxicity in the rat. *Hear Res* 1996; 102:90–98.
34. Nicotera TM, Hu BH, Henderson D. The caspase pathway in noise-induced apoptosis of the chinchilla cochlea. *J Assoc Res Otolaryngol* 2003; 4(4):466–477.
35. Seidman MD. Effects of dietary restriction and antioxidants on presbyacusis. *Laryngoscope* 2000; 110:727–738.
36. Gates GA, Couropmitree NN, Myers RH. Genetic associations in age-related hearing thresholds. *Arch Otolaryngol Head Neck Surg* 1999; 125(6):654–659.
37. Johnson KR, Zheng QY, Erway LC. A major gene affecting age-related hearing loss is common to at least ten inbred strains of mice. *Genomics* 2000; 70(2):171–180.
38. Jimenez AM, Stagner BB, Martin GK, Lonsbury-Martin BL. Susceptibility of DPOAEs to sound overexposure in inbred mice with AHL. *J Assoc Res Otolaryngol* 2001; 2(3):233–245.
39. Ballanchanda B. Cerumen and the ear canal secretory system. In: Ballanchanda B, ed. *Introduction to the Human Ear Canal*. San Diego: Singular Publishing Group, 1995: 181–201.
40. Novak R. Considerations for selecting and fitting of amplification for geriatric adults. In: Sandlin RE, ed. *Textbook of Hearing Aid Amplification*. San Diego, CA: Singular Publishing Group, 2000: 571–606.
41. Gleitman R, Ballachanda B, Goldstein. Incidence of cerumen impaction in general adult population. *Hear J* 1992; 45:28–32.
42. Willott J. *Aging and the Auditory System*. San Diego: Singular Publishing Group; 1991.
43. Otte J, Schunknecht HF, Kerr AG. Ganglion cell populations in normal and pathological human cochleae. Implications for cochlear implantation. *Laryngoscope* 1978; 88:1231–1246.
44. Suzuka Y, Schuknecht HF. Retrograde cochlear neuronal degeneration in human subjects. *Acta Otolaryngol Suppl* 1988; 450:1–20.
45. Pauler M, Schuknecht HF, Thornton AR. Correlative studies of cochlear neuronal loss with speech discrimination and pure-tone thresholds. *Arch Otorhinolaryngol* 1986; 243(3):200–206.
46. Crandell C, Henoch M, Dunkerson K. A review of speech perception and aging: Some implications for aural rehabilitation. *J Am Acad Rehabil Audiol* 1991; 24:121–133.
47. Bellis TJ, Wilber LA. Effects of aging and gender on interhemispheric function. *J Speech Lang Hear Res* 2001; 44(2):246–263.
48. Wiley TL, Cruickshanks KJ, Nondahl DM, Tweed TS, Klein R, Klein BE. Aging and word recognition in competing message. *J Am Acad Audiol* 1998; 9(3):191–198.
49. Stach BA, Spretnjak ML, Jerger J. The prevalence of central presbyacusis in a clinical population. *J Am Acad Audiol* 1990; 1(2):109–115.
50. Martin JS, Jerger JF. Some effects of aging on central auditory processing. *J Rehabil Res Dev* 2005; 42(4 Suppl 2):25–44.
51. Gordon-Salant S. Hearing loss and aging: new research findings and clinical implications. *J Rehabil Res Dev* 2005; 42(4 Suppl 2):9–24.
52. Wingfield A, Tun PA. Spoken language comprehension in older adults: Interactions between sensory and cognitive change in normal aging. *Sem Hear* 2001; 22:287–301.
53. Gordon-Salant S, Fitzgibbons P. Selected cognitive factors and speech recognition performance among young and elderly listeners. *J Speech Lang Hear Res* 1997; 40:423–431.

54. Bentler R. Effectiveness of directional microphones and noise reduction schemes in hearing aids: a systematic review of the evidence. *J Am Acad Audiol* 2005; 16(7):473–484.
55. Jerger J, Chmiel R, Florin E, Pirozzolo F, Wilson N. Comparison of conventional amplification and an assistive listening device in elderly persons. *Ear Hear* 1996; 17:490–504.
56. Gatehouse S, Naylor G, Elberling C. Benefits from hearing aids in relation to the interaction between the user and the environment. *Int J Audiol* 2003; 42(Suppl 1):S77–S85.
57. Pichora-Fuller MK, Singh G. Effects of age on auditory and cognitive processing: Implications for hearing aid fitting and audiologic rehabilitation. *Trends Amplif* 2006; 10(1):29–59.
58. Greenwald R, Jerger J. Aging affects hemispheric asymmetry on a competing speech task. *J Am Acad Audiol* 2001; 12:167–173.
59. Byrne D. Clinical issues and options in binaural hearing aid fitting. *Ear Hear* 1981; 2:187–193.
60. Walden T, Walden B. Unilateral versus bilateral amplification for adults with impaired hearing. *J Am Acad Audiol* 2005; 16:574–584.
61. Boothroyd A. Hearing aid accessories for adults: the remote FM microphone. *Ear Hear* 2004; 25(1):22–33.
62. Chisolm T, McArdle R, Abrams H, Noe C. Goals and outcomes of FM use by adults. *Hear J* 2004; 57:28–35.
63. Russell E, Burns A. Presentation and clinical management of dementia. In: Tallis R, Fillitt H, Brockelhurst J, eds. *Brockelhurst's Textbook of Geriatric Medicine and Gerontology*. London: Churchill Livingstone, 1999: 727–740.
64. Uhlmann R, Larson E, Rees T, Koespell T, Duckert L. Relationship of hearing impairment to dementia and cognitive dysfunction in older adults. *J Am Med Assoc* 1989; 261: 1916–1919.
65. Grimes A. Auditory changes. In: Lubinski R, ed. *Dementia and Communication*. San Diego: Singular Publishing Group, 1995: 47–69.
66. Kricos PB. Audiologic management of older adults with hearing loss and compromised cognitive/psychoacoustic auditory processing capabilities. *Trends Amplif* 2006; 10(1):1–8.
67. Mulrow C, Tuley M, Aguilar C. Sustained benefits of hearing aids. *J Speech Lang Hear Res* 1992; 35:1402–1405.
68. Wallhagen M, Strawbridge W, Shema S. Impact of self-assessed hearing loss on a spouse: A longitudinal analysis of couples. *J Geront Soc Sci* 2004; 59:S190–S196.
69. Kaplan H. Benefits and limitations of amplification and speechreading for the elderly. In: Orlans H, ed. *Adjustment to Adult Hearing Loss*. San Diego, CA: Singular Publishing Group, 1991: 85–98.
70. Webb L, Schreiner J, Asmuth M. Maintaining interaction skills. In: Huntley R, Helfer K, eds. *Communication Skills in Later Life*. Boston, MA: Butterworth Heinemann, 1995: 159–179.
71. Cacciatore F, Abete P, Napoli C, Marciano E, Triassi M, Rengo F. Quality of life determinants and hearing function in an elderly population. *Gerontology* 1999; 45:323–328.
72. Hession C. Hearing loss and aging: Psychosocial aspects and implications for rehabilitation. *Texas J Audiol Speech Path* 1991; 17(2):10–13.
73. Meadow-Orlans K. Social and psychological effects of hearing loss in adulthood: A literature review. In: Orlans H, ed. *Adjustment to Adult Hearing Loss*. San Diego: Singular Publishing Group, 1991: 35–57.
74. Pray J. Parallel reactions in hearing loss in later years. An Elderhostel Guide and Course Supplement. Washington, DC: Gallaudet University, 1996.
75. Ventry I, Weinstein B. The Hearing Handicap Inventory for the Elderly: A new tool. *Ear Hear* 1982; 3(3):128–134.
76. Beck RL. The forgotten family. *SHHH* 1991; 12(1):7–9.
77. Newman C, Weinstein B. Judgments of perceived hearing handicap by hearing-impaired elderly men and their spouses. *J Acad Rehabil Audiol* 1996; 19:109–115.
78. Quinn KS. Self spouse and audiologist evaluation of hearing impairment and hearing handicap in a sample of older people (dissertation): University of Michigan; 1986.

79. Palmer C. Improvement of hearing function. In: Huntley RA, Helfer KS, eds. *Communication in Later Life*. Boston, MA: Butterworth-Heinemann, 1995: 181–221.

80. Hooker K, Shifren K. Psychological aspects of aging. In: Huntley RA, Helfer KS, eds. *Communication in Later Life*. Boston, MA: Butterworth-Heinemann, 1995: 99–126.

81. Pray J. Aging and hearing loss: Patterns of coping with the effects of late onset hearing loss among persons 60 and older and their spouses/significant others.(dissertation): The Union Institute;1992.

82. Gould R. *Transformations*. New York: Simon & Schuster, 1978.

83. Erikson E, Erikson J, Kivnick H. *Vital Involvement in Old Age*. New York: W. Norton, 1986.

84. Maurer J, Rupp R. *Hearing and Aging*. New York: Grune and Stratton, 1979.

85. Glass L. Psychosocial aspects of hearing loss in adulthood. In: Orlans H, ed. *Adjustment to Adult Hearing Loss*. San Diego, CA: Singular Publishing Group, 1991: 167–178.

86. Schlesinger HS. The psychology of hearing loss. In: Orlans H, ed. *Adjustment to Adult Hearing Loss*. San Diego, CA: College-Hill Press, 1985: 99–118.

87. Perlstein R. Mature market report. Mature Market Report, Inc. Atlanta, GA: College-Hill Press, 1990.

88. Ross M. Why people won't wear hearing aids. *Hear Rehabil Quart* 1992; 17(2).

89. Harvey MA. *Psychotherapy with Deaf and Hard of Hearing Persons: A systemic model*. 2nd ed. Mahweh, NJ: Lawrence Erlbaum Associates, 2003.

90. Weinstein B. *Geriatric Audiology*. New York: Thieme, 2000.

91. Hooyman N, Kivak H. *Social Gerontology: A Multidisciplinary Perspective*, 5th ed. Boston: Allyn & Bacon, 1999.

92. Brennan M, Heiser D. *Spiritual Assessment and Intervention Among Older Adults*. Binghamton, NY: Haworth Pastoral Press, 2005.

93. Brennan M. Spirituality and religiousness predict adaptation to vision loss among middle-age and older adults. *Int J Psy Rel* 2004;14(3):193–214.

94. Kubler-Ross F. *On Death and Dying*. New York: McMillan, 1969.

95. Carabellese C, Appolonio I, Rozzini R, Bianchetti A, Frisoni G, Frattola L, et al. Sensory impairment and quality of life in a community elderly population. *J Am Geriatr Soc* 1993; 41:401–407.

96. Maggi S, Minicicuci N, Martini A, Langlois J, Siviero P, Pavan, et al. Prevalence rates of hearing impairment and comorbid conditions in older people: The Veneto Study. *J Am Geriatr Soc* 1998; 46:1069–1074.

97. Strawbridge W, Wallhagen M, Shema S, Kaplan G. Negative consequences of hearing impairment in old age: A longitudinal analysis. *Gerontologist* 2000; 40:320–326.

98. Bazargan M, Baker R, Bazargan H. Sensory impairments and subjective well being among aged African American persons. *J Geront* 2001; 56B(5):268–278.

99. Almeida O. Clinical and cognitive diversity of psychotic states arising in late life-late paraphrenia. (dissertation). University of London, England; 1993.

100. Appollonio I, Carabellese C, Frattola L, Trabucchi M. Effects of sensory aids on the quality of life and mortality of elderly people: a multivariate analysis. *Age Aging* 1996; 25(2):89–96.

101. Kreeger J, Raulin M, Grace J, Priest B. Effect of hearing enhancement on mental status ratings in geriatric psychiatric patients. *Am J Psychiatry* 1995; 152:629–631.

102. Bazargan M, Barbe A. The effects of depression, health status, and stressful life events on self-reported memory problems among status, and stressful life-events on self-reported memory problems among aged Blacks. *Int J Aging Human Dev* 1994; 38:151–162.

103. Lindenberger U, Baltes PB. Sensory functioning and intelligence in old age: A strong connection. *Psychol Aging* 1994; 9:339–355.

104. Mulrow C, Aguilar C, Endicott J, Velez R, Tuley MR,Charlip WS, et al. Association between hearing impairment and the quality of life of elderly individuals. *J Am Geriatr Soc* 1990; 38(1):45–50.

105. Scherer M, Frisina D. Characteristics associated with marginal hearing loss and subjective well-being among a sample of older adults. *J Rehabil Res Dev* 1998; 35:420–426.

106. Resnick H, Fries B, Vergrugge L. Windows to their world: the effect of sensory impairment on social engagement and activity in nursing home residents. *J Gerontol* 1997; 528:S135–S144.
107. Palmore F. Normal aging ii: Reports from the Duke longitudinal studies. Durham, NC: Duke University Press, 1974.
108. Butler R. *Why Survive? Being Old in America*. New York: Harper & Row, 1975.
109. Datan N, Ginsberg L. *Life Span Developmental Psychology: Normative Life Crises*. New York: Academic Press, 1975.
110. Rosow I. Social contact of the aging self. *Gerontologist* 1973; 13:82–87.
111. Rosow I. *Socialization to Old Age*. Berkeley, CA: University of California Press, 1974.
112. Maas H, Kuypers J. *From Thirty to Seventy*. San Francisco: Jossey-Bass, 1974.
113. Orr J. Aging, catastrophe, and moral reasoning. In: McKee P, ed. *Philosophical Foundations of Gerontology*. New York: Human Sciences Press, 1982: 243–260.
114. Wax T. The hearing impaired aged: Double jeopardy or double challenge? *Gallaudet Today* 1982; 12(2):3–7.
115. Markides K. Minority aging. In: Riley M, Hess B, Bond K, eds. *Aging in Society: Selected review of recent research*. Hillsdale, NJ: Lawrence Erlbaum Associates, 1983: 115–137.
116. Calhoun DW, Lipman A. The disabled. In: Palmore ED, ed. *Handbook on the Aged in the United States*. Westport, CT: Greenwood Press, 1984: 311–322.
117. Goffman F. *Stigma: Notes on the management of spoiled identity*. Englewood Cliffs, NJ: Prentice-Hall, 1963.
118. Watson WH, Maxwell RJ. *Human Aging and Dying: A study in sociocultural gerontology*. New York: St Martin's Press, 1977.
119. Fadiman A. *The Spirit Catches You and You Fall Down*. New York: Noonday Press, 1997.
120. Schow RL, Balsara NR, Whitcomb CJ, Smedley TC. Aural rehabilitation by ASHA audiologists: 1980–1990. *Am J Audiol* 1993;2(3):28–37.
121. Carmen R. Survey of audiologists from an online questionnaire. (Accessed June 5, 2003, at http://www.audiologyonline.com).
122. Prendergast SG, Kelley LA. Aural rehabilitation services: Survey reports who offers which ones and how often. *Hear J* 2002;55(9):30–35.
123. National Institute on Deafness and Other Communication Disorders. Cochlear Implants (Accessed December 12, 2006, at http://www.nidcd.nih.gov).
124. Kaplan H, Bally S, Brandt F, Busacco D, Pray J. The communication self-assessment scales for older adults (CSOA). *J Am Acad Audiol* 1997;8(3):203–217.
125. Schow R, Nerbonne M. Assessment of hearing handicap by nursing home residents and staff. *J Rehabil Audiol* 1977;10:2–12.
126. Compton-Conley C, Bernstein C. Hearing assistance technology needs assessment profile (HATNAP): A web-based system designed to enable consumers to navigate through their own receptive communication needs assessment. The 3rd International Adult Aural Rehabilitation Conference; 2005 May 9-12; Portland, Maine.
127. Compton C. Assistive technology for deaf and hard-of-hearing people. In: Alpiner J, McCarthy P, eds. *Rehabilitative Audiology: Children and adults*. Baltimore, MD: Lippincott, Williams and Wilkins, 2002: 501–544.
128. Compton C. Assistive technology for deaf and hard-of-hearing people. In: Alpiner J, McCarthy P, eds. *Rehabilitative Audiology: Children and adults*. Baltimore, MD: Williams and Wilkins, 1993: 441–468.
129. Vaughn G, Lightfoot R. ALDS pioneers: Past and present: Part III: ALDS triad-service, education and research. *Hear Instr* 1987; 38:4–12.
130. Palmer C, Garstecki D. A computer spreadsheet for locating assistive devices. *J Acad Rehabil Audiol* 1988; 21:158–175.
131. Ross M. Hearing assistance technology: making a world of difference. *Hear J* 2004; 57:12–17.
132. Thibodeau L. Plotting beyond the audiogram to the Telegram, a new assessment tool. *Hear J* 2004; 57:46–51.

133. Compton C. Selecting what's best for the individual. In: Tyler R, Schum D, eds. *Assistive Devices for Persons with Hearing Impairment*. Boston: Allyn & Bacon, 1995: 224–250.
134. Dillon H. *Hearing Aids*. New York: Thieme, 2001.
135. Bakke MH, Levitt H, Ross M, Erickson F. Large area assistive listening systems (ALS): Review and recommendations: Final report to United States Architectural and Transportation Barriers Compliance Board (U.S. Access Board). Lexington School for the Deaf/Center for the Deaf, Rehabilitation Engineering Research Center on Hearing Enhancement. New York, 1999 (Accessed January 8, 2007 at http://www.hearingresearch.org/ publications_and_presentations.htm).
136. Dillon H, Lovegrove R. Single-microphone noise reduction systems for hearing aids: a review and an evaluation. In: Studebaker GA, Hochberg I, eds. *Acoustical Factors Affecting Hearing Aid Performance*. Needham Heights, MA: Allyn & Bacon, 1993: 353–372.
137. UK Cochlear Implant Study Group. Criteria of candidacy for unilateral cochlear implantation in postlingually deafened adults I: theory and measures of effectiveness. *Ear Hear* 2004;25(4):310–335.
138. Francis HW, Chee N, Yeagle J, Cheng A, Niparko JN. Impact of cochlear implants on the functional health status of older adults. *Laryngoscope* 2002; 112:1482–1488.
139. Leal M., Shin Y., Laborde M., Calmels M., Verges S., Lugardon S, et al. Music perception in adult cochlear implant recipients. *Acta Oto-Laryngologica* 2003; 123(7):826–835.
140. Waltzman S. Cochlear implants and evolving technology. State of the Science Conference on Assisitive Technologies for People with Hearing Loss; 2001 May 11; Graduate Center, City University of New York, NY.
141. Plomp R. Auditory handicap of hearing impairment and the limited benefit of hearing aids. *J Acoust Soc Am* 1978;63:533–549.
142. Nabelek AK. Communication in noisy and reverberant environments. In: Studebaker GA, Hochberg I, eds. *Acoustical Factors Affecting Hearing Aid Performance*. Needham Heights, MA: Allyn & Bacon, 1993: 15–28.
143. Stickney G, Zeng F, Litovsky R, Assmann P. Cochlear implant speech recognition with speech maskers. *J Acoust Soc Am* 2004; 116(2):1081–1091.
144. Lesner S. Candidacy and management of assistive listening devices: special needs of the elderly. *Int J Audiol* 2003; 42:2S68–2S76.
145. Mann W, Hurren D, Tomita M, Charvat B. The relationship of functional dependence to assistive device use of elderly persons living at home. *J Appl Gerontol* 1995; 14:225–247.
146. National Center for Health Statistics. Current Estimates from the National Health Interview Survey, 1989. Vital and Health Statistics, 10, Hyattsville, MD: National Center for Health Statistics, 1990.
147. Brooks DN. Factors relating to the under-use of postaural hearing aids. *Br J Audiol* 1985; 19(3):211–217.
148. Lubinski R. Perspectives on aging and communication. In: Lubinski R, Higginbotham D, eds. *Communication Technologies for the Elderly: Vision, Hearing, and Speech*. San Diego: Singular Publishing Group, 1997: 1–21.
149. Riemer-Reiss M, Wacker R. Factors associated with assistive technology discontinuance among individuals with disabilities. *J Rehabil* 2000; 66:44–59.
150. Ross M. Hearing assistive technology training; University of Florida, 2006.
151. Surr RK, Schuchman GI, Montgomery AA. Factors influencing use of hearing aids. *Arch Otolaryngol* 1978; 104:732–736.
152. Brooks DN. Hearing aid use and the effects of counseling. *Aust J Audiol* 1979; 1(1):1–6.
153. Smaldino SE, Smaldino JJ. The influence of aural rehabilitation and cognitive style discourse on the perception of hearing handicap. *J Am Acad Rehabil Audiol* 1988; 21:57–64.
154. Abrams HB, Hnath-Chisolm T, Guerreiro SM, Ritterman SI. The effects of intervention strategy on self-perception of hearing handicap. *Ear Hear* 1992; 13(5):371–377.
155. Kricos PB, Holmes AE. Efficacy of audiologic rehabilitation for older adults. *J Am Acad Audiol* 1996; 7(4):219–229.

156. Northern J, Meadows-Beyer C. Reducing hearing aid returns through patient education. *Audiol Today* 1999; 11(2):10–13.
157. Hawkins D. Effectiveness of counseling-based adult group aural rehabilitation programs: a systematic review of the evidence. *J Am Acad Audiol* 2005; 16(7):485–493.
158. Sweetow R, Henderson-Sabes. The case for LACE (Listening and Communication Enhancement). *Hear J* 2004; 57(3): 32–40.

Chapter 8
Falls, Fall Prevention, and Fall Detection Technologies

Prabhu Rajendran, Amy Corcoran, Bruce Kinosian, and Majd Alwan

8.1 Necessity

Over one-third of elders 65-year old and over fall each year, nearly 13 million fall a year. Nearly half are a recurrent fall, and nearly 10% of falls result in serious injuries. Over 64% of injuries to patients 70 years old and over occur because of a fall, which included 13,000 deaths in 2002 [1]. A 4-year prospective cohort study of a trauma registry found that of those 65 years old and over ($n = 333$), falls were the mechanism of injury in 48% ($n = 159$). Of those who fall, 47% suffered soft tissue/skin injuries, whereas 47% head/neck injuries, 23% chest injuries, and 27% pelvis/extremity injuries. Those who suffered moderate to severe injuries, such as hip fractures or head traumas, had reduced mobility and independence afterwards. Closed-head injuries were found to be the most common cause of death [2].

The cost of caring for elderly after a fall is substantial, although estimates vary. Some suggest that fall-related injuries account for 6% of all medical expenditures in the USA [3–5]. The Centers for Disease Control (CDC) cites a more discrete approach that estimates the direct cost of fall-related injuries in 2000 at $19 billion [5]. In 2003, approximately 1.8 million persons 65 years old and greater were treated in emergency departments for fall-related injuries, with more than 421,000 hospitalized [1]. In community dwellers who sustain a fall and hip fracture, up to 25% remain institutionalized, and 15–20% are dead at 1 year. More than 50% become dependent for lower extremity tasks such as walking, climbing stairs, and rising from sitting [6].

Location of where the elderly most commonly fall is important in preventing and detecting falls. About 35–40% of community-dwelling elders fall annually [7]. In nursing home facilities and hospitals, the fall rate is three times higher in those older than 65 years old when compared with those living in the community, about 1.5 falls per bed annually in institutions [3,4]. The risk of falling increases with age.

Majd Alwan
Director, Center for Aging Services Technologies (CAST), 2519 Connecticut Ave. NW, Washington, DC 20008-1520
e-mail: malwan@agingtech.org

From: *Aging Medicine, Eldercare Technology for Clinical Practitioners,*
Edited by: M. Alwan and R. Felder © Humana Press, Totowa, NJ

For example, a 5-year prospective study of an active ambulatory institutionalized population of adults over the age of 65 years revealed an annual fall rate of 668 incidents per 1000, with an increase in frequency for successive age groups above the age of 75 years [8]. In another recent study of 121 elderly over 3 years, the incidence of falls at group dwellings for patient's with dementia was twice the rates of the senior housing apartments and older people's homes in Sweden. Of the 428 falls that occurred, 118 lead to at least one injury without a significant difference among the three types of housing. Falls in the group dwelling, primarily patients with dementia, were more frequently associated with rising/sitting down (46% of 69 falls), as opposed to walking in the old people's homes (56% of 156 falls) [9].

8.2 Types of Fall Prevention

Interventions have been used to reduce the burden of falls at several stages of prevention: primary (preventing a fall), secondary (detecting a fall early and preventing/mitigating injury from a fall), and tertiary (reducing morbidity from fall-related injuries). We briefly review the general framework for primary prevention, which has been extensively reviewed elsewhere [4, 7]. In the remainder of this chapter, we will focus on two aspects of secondary prevention: limiting morbidity from a fall by reducing the impact of the fall by protecting the faller, and by detecting a fall early and reducing response time for rescue or intervention.

8.2.1 Primary Prevention

Effective fall primary prevention programs rely on the identification of intrinsic and extrinsic risk factors associated with potential falls and fall injuries. Programs then make a decision on the appropriate strategies for individual and environmental intervention to prevent future falls. Some of the common intrinsic factors that increase the incidence of the falls, as cited in various systematic reviews on this topic, include visual deficits, stroke, arthritis, orthostatic hypotension, acute illnesses, unsteady gait, poor balance, cognitive impairment, and incontinence [10–12]. Previous falls, associated with intrinsic risk factors, are an additional, potent risk factor. The extrinsic factors include medications and various environmental factors such as loose carpets, throw-rugs, doorsteps, unsafe stairways, bathtubs without handles, and poor lighting besides other factors [13, 14]. A number of intervention studies, focused on addressing individual risk factors or multiple risk factors have been conducted over the past two decades. Recent reviews have found risk reductions of 14–39% in several studies when a multi-factorial risk assessment with targeted management is implemented through health care providers [15, 16], and an estimated risk reduction of 29–49% using specific balance or strength exercise programs (including Tai Chi) for community-dwelling elders without any health care intervention or risk stratification [15]. The specific intervention components that are most successful include medication review and reduction, balance and gait training, muscle-strengthening exercises, evaluating for orthostatic hypotension, home-safety evaluation and modification, and focusing on the management of cardiovascular and chronic medical problems [15, 17]. Using appropriate assistive devices such as mobility aids (walkers, wheelchairs) can also help prevent future falls. In combination with other fall prevention strategies, the subjects in the higher risk population must be encouraged to participate in individual and/or group exercise programs, which are based on the individual's functional ability, to help improve the person's performance, strength, and balance. Targeting these interventions to those at greater risk of falling is important. Risk-screening methods are aimed at identifying fall-prone individuals. Morse fall scale [18] and Heslin fall scale [19] are two of the most popular screening tools used to identify a higher risk population and specific risk factors.

Recommending restraints to prevent falls, contrary to old beliefs, has been proven to be one of the least effective prevention strategies. In fact, several studies have found that restraints actually increase the severity of falls [20]. Various alternatives to restraints, such as medication modifications, low beds, specialized positioning devices, alert systems, and more, have been suggested in the literature [21]. In a retrospective case control study of 929 records of first time fallers who were restrained, those restrained were 14 times more likely to fall than those who were not restrained [22]. Besides increasing the severity of falls, using restraints may also result in loss of dignity and independence, increased agitation, and depression. Similarly, some medications used as "chemical restraints" (such as several psychotropics and benzodiazepines) are prominent among those medications associated with increased risk of falling [13].

In addition to the numerous physical and cognitive conditions that result in the increased incidence of falls, psychological effects of falls and fear of falling are independent risk factors for future falls [23]. Individuals may restrict their mobility unnecessarily after a fall, which may lead to social isolation, further degradation in the physical condition, and increased risk of falls. A person's confidence or self efficacy to perform daily activities without falling has been shown to be closely related to actual performance. Self efficacy, thus, is an important target for interventions to the fall-risk population.

8.2.1.1 Fall Watch Alarm Technologies

Systematic reviews of the literature have also revealed that most of the common fall prevention technologies used in the institutional setting like pressure-based bed alarms and identification bracelets are not effective in reducing the incidence of falls [24, 25]. The approach is to alert staff when an "at risk" person starts to rise and walk, which may reduce response time. However, their effectiveness in reducing falls is dependent upon other factors, such as setting and staffing. For example, in a small group home with a low client–caregiver ratio, the chance that an alarm will

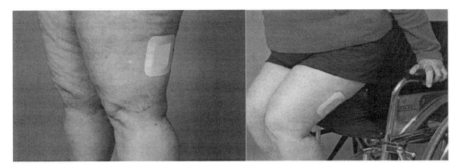

Fig. 8.1 NOC-Watch device (published with permission)

result in a response before a fall is substantially greater than in a large, understaffed facility. Such devices, by themselves, have been proven insufficient to reduce falls, but may increase awareness of staff and providers of those at risk. An example of this type of motion-alarm device is the NOC-watch device [26], which consists of a credit card size device contained within an adhesive "patch" worn directly on the thigh continuously for many days. The device can also be incorporated into clothing such as pants or hip protectors, although the device's usefulness is then limited to the hours the outer garments are worn. The patch is small, wireless, disposable, waterproof, shockproof, and unobtrusive. The NOC-watch transmitter inside the adhesive pouch sends a signal from the patient's thigh to a receiver in the patient's room when the patient gets out of bed or wheelchair unassisted. This event is indicated by a patient's leg becoming weight-bearing, which occurs within a cone-shaped area approximately 60–70 degrees below horizontal. The device reliably detects high fall risk behavior and can alert both the patient and the caregiver in time for preemptive action without generating false alarms (Figure 8.1).

This device is recommended, in a clinical setting, for subjects who are more prone to falls as indicated by a high fall risk score on Fall Risk Assessment (FRA), which is based on various risk factors including vision, recent fall history, medications, and ambulation ability. One clinical study conducted to measure the efficacy of the device indicated that wearing NOC-watch resulted in a 91% reduction of falls in a nursing home setting; however, as mentioned above, the performance largely depends on staffing level and thus response time, so has limited generalizability. The device also appeared to be very effective in reducing fall risk behavior in the high-risk dementia population, who have particular difficulty remembering not to ambulate or calling for assistance before attempting to ambulate. Acceptance of the device by staff and patients appeared to be high, and no adverse effects on skin integrity were noted during the length of the study. The cost of a NOC-watch device is estimated to be around $2 per day for the patches that are attached directly to the patient's skin. The cost significantly decreases for the versions that are implemented in the clothing as the lifetime of patch increases considerably [26].

When setting and staffing are not conducive to preventing falls, such devices function as a means to reduce injury.

8.2.2 Secondary Prevention

8.2.2.1 Hip Protectors

Studies have shown that secondary intervention devices such as hip protectors are effective in reducing the effect of falls [27], but they are usually met with high patient resistance to routine wear partially because of the added bulk under clothes and perceptions of older patients [28]. Fractures are reduced among those who wear protectors while they do so, but the overall individual fracture risk has often not been reduced in studies, because of the substantial time when elders do not wear the protectors. In several recent meta-analyses, hip protectors have been found to offer a small reduction in fractures in the nursing home setting because of higher enforced compliance, but not in the community setting [28, 29] (Figure 8.2).

8.2.2.2 Safe Floors

Streit and Cavanaugh at Pennsylvania State University, developed and validated a finite element model (FEM) for use in the design of a flooring system that would provide a stable walking surface during normal locomotion but would also deform elastically under higher loads, such as those resulting from falls. A floor was constructed using prototype floor tiles [30]. The study demonstrated that a floor can be designed that deflects minimally during walking but that will reduce the peak force on the femoral neck during a fall-related impact by 15.2% [31]. However, the floor was costly to manufacture and some institutional building codes related to flooring material in assisted living facilities were important barriers to further applications and field testing.

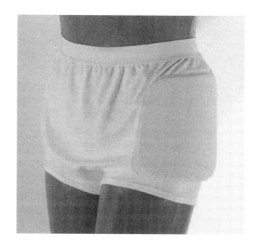

Fig. 8.2 Hip protector from AliMed® (image is copyrighted property of AliMed®)

8.2.2.3 Fall Detector Types

The medical outcome of a fall may be largely dependent upon the response and rescue time. Hence, reliable fall detection and notification is essential in independent living facilities. Fall event detection followed by immediate reporting to caregivers certainly could improve health outcome by initiating faster caregiver response and facilitating appropriate medical care or evaluation.

Fall detectors, both commercially available and under research, can generally be classified under one or a combination of the following four broad categories:

1. User-activated alarms and pendants;
2. Automatic wearable fall detectors;
3. Video monitoring-based fall detectors;
4. Floor Vibration-based fall detectors.

User-Activated Alarms and Pendants

These devices, generally, require the user to manually activate an alarm button, which is appropriate for those cognitively intact older persons. Usually the alarm button is on a pendent or a bracelet integrated with a wireless transmitter or transceiver, to be pressed in the event of falling. When pressed, the alarm button wirelessly activates a medical alert unit that is connected to the telephone. The medical alert system then calls the monitoring center dedicated for medical emergency alarm monitoring. An attendant in the monitoring center will immediately speak to the subscriber. The attendant then alerts the subscriber's personal responders, which may include family members, friends or emergency services depending on the attendant's discernment of the subscriber's condition. A number of Eldercare facilities and Community Alarm Centers (i.e., Philips Life Line, BLEEP, Lifefone, MedicalAlarm.com) offer such services for a nominal monthly monitoring fee (Figure 8.3).

Although such fall alarms are simple and low-cost (in terms of purchase price), they are not effective for falls associated with the loss of consciousness or if the subject was unable to activate the alarm because of trauma, pain, or other reasons. Manual activation may not occur in cases of elderly adults with dementia, as the user may forget to activate the device. Such devices rely on the premise that the user is wearing the device all the time so as to activate them when needed. Nonetheless, users may take the device off, in the shower or in bed for example, and hence they may fall while not wearing the device.

Automatic Wearable Fall Detectors

Various automatic fall detectors that do not require manual activation have been designed to overcome some of the common drawbacks of the user-activated alarms. Automatic detectors are commonly available in the wearable form. Human falls are generally characterized by an impact on the floor followed by the near horizontal orientation of the faller. Most of the automatic fall detectors are designed to detect

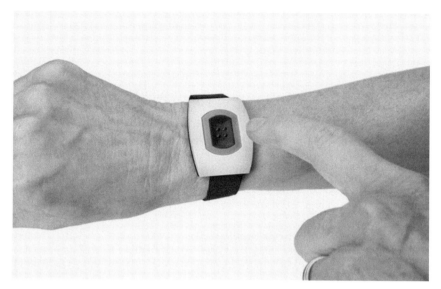

Fig. 8.3 Philips Lifeline Slimline(tm) Personal Help Button (Copyright © Lifeline is a registered trademark of Philips)

one or both of these effects [32]. Accelerometers are employed in the design to detect an impact whereas tilt sensors and/or gyroscopes are used to determine the orientation of the faller after the impact and tilt transitions during the event of fall. There are many designs available under this category depending on the locations for wearing the fall detector. The common locations for wearing fall detectors include chest (neck pendant), hips or waist (belt or pocket), wrist or forearm (bracelet or watchstrap), knee or thigh (strap or stocking). Conspicuous wearable fall detectors, such as the ones we will describe below, may be perceived by the users as a stigma labeling them as fallers among their peers.

One of the popular commercial brands of fall detector in this category is developed by Tunstall Group Ltd. Although small enough to be carried ready for use in a handbag, wallet, or purse, this device must be worn on the body if it is to detect a fall. The company's website (www.tunstall.co.uk) suggests that the device must be worn where it will receive the shock associated with a fall. Whilst there is no specific ideal location for the detector, it should always be worn at or above the waist. Also, the Fall Detector must be worn where it will assume the inclination of the body following a fall. Provided the device is fixed to clothing at or above the waist, it will measure the body's inclination within an acceptable tolerance of 10–15 degrees and will detect more than 90% of all falls onto a horizontal floor. However, an alarm may not be automatically triggered immediately following a fall when the fall is incomplete and the faller's torso does not assume a horizontal inclination. An example is when a slump to the ground is interrupted by an item of furniture or the stairs. Under these circumstances, the fall detector would be activated by the impact but may not sense that the person has fallen to the ground. In the unlikely event that the fall detector is not automatically activated, the wearer can use the manual alarm button in the device to call for help.

The chest wearable fall detector currently being developed at Seoul National University [33] aims to accomplish real-time ambulatory monitoring of falls in fall-prone populations, including older adults. The system is composed of a real-time sensing circuit and a two-way communication circuit. The sensing circuit comprises a tri-axial accelerometer, gyroscope (Murata, ENC-03J, ±400°/s), and a tilt sensor. The communication circuit comprises Bluetooth transceiver and Microcontroller. The communication circuit is integrated with a sensing circuit for real-time monitoring/communication between the elderly user and a caregiver. In this system, the accelerometer measures kinetic force in each of the three axes, whereas the gyroscope estimates posture transition and tilt sensor detects whether the subject is supine or standing. Data obtained from the sensors are then transmitted to data acquisition (DAQ) program through Bluetooth Module, which a caregiver (for example a physician) can use to monitor elderly people at real time. A fall is detected when the acceleration of the subject changes rapidly followed by a change in the orientation of the user to greater than 70 degrees, which is typical in human falls. Following this, a timer is initiated for 10 s during which the system looks for acceleration variations above a pre-set threshold. A fall alarm will be generated by the system when there are no significant acceleration variations during this period. Of a total of 123 trials conducted to test the performance of the fall detector in a controlled laboratory set up, the system succeeded 119 times and failed four times. Although the system could detect the forward and backward falls with impressive accuracy and repeatability, it was observed that only four of the 10 emulated sideway falls could be detected, which may be due to positioning of the sensors at the chest.

Researchers at the Swiss Federal Institute of Technology developed Speedy [34], a first prototype of a fall detector integrated into a wrist watch. Small, easy to handle, and inconspicuous, it is aimed at elders living alone at home or in senior housing. Speedy will alert relatives or a call center through a wireless link to a local telephone central when the user presses the incorporated alarm button or if he/ she falls and loses consciousness. The authors point out that the other common fall detectors, generally attached to a belt around the hip, are less comfortable and inadequate to be worn during the sleep which results in the inability of such detectors to monitor the critical phase of getting up from the bed; knowing that falls while getting out of bed are prevalent among elders because of postural hypotension. However, the major disadvantage of integrating the fall detector in a wrist watch is the relative complexity in the determination of falls as the arms have six degrees of freedom (as arms can both move and rotate). The main components of Speedy are two accelerometers, a Microcontroller, and a wireless RF-Link to the base station. A fall is detected when a high velocity toward the ground is followed by an impact within 3 s. After the impact, the general activity will be observed for 60 s. If during this interval at least 40 s of inactivity are recorded, Speedy will generate an audible alarm. The wearer can then deactivate the alarm by pushing on the button for 1 s. If the wearer does not respond to the alarm tone by pressing the button, the alarm will

Fig. 8.4 Speedy—A fall detector integrated in a wrist watch (Source Acknowledgement: thomas.degen@ieee.org)

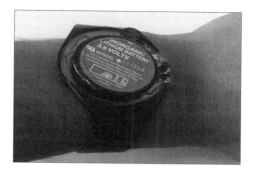

be transmitted wireless to the base station, which will then alert a call center. The fall tests conducted to evaluate the reliability of fall detection showed that Speedy could detect falls with an overall accuracy of 65%. The fall detection results were poor in the backwards and sideways fall scenarios (58 and 45%, respectively). The system, however exhibited impressive specificity (i.e., low false alarm rate) (Figure 8.4).

Worn devices generally have the advantage of being small, light-weight, easy-to-use, relatively low cost, and of being available on a "plug and play" basis for anyone who has a community alarm telephone. However, they can only perform their function correctly and reliably if they are worn correctly at all times when the subject is up and about.

Video monitoring-Based Fall Detectors

Ideally, these devices are required to be placed in each and every room where the occurrence of falls needs to be detected. These devices track the resident using cameras installed at vantage locations and attempt to detect a fall event based on image-processing algorithms that are designed to identify unusual inactivity, which is more likely to follow an event of fall. The fall detectors under this category are passive in the sense that they generally do not require the user to wear any device. Universities worldwide are conducting research in the development of video analysis-based fall detection systems to explore the various possible design variations in image-processing algorithms and monitoring/transmission systems.

The UbiSense project [35], at the Imperial College London, aims to develop an unobtrusive health-monitoring system for the elderly by using embedded smart vision techniques to detect changes in posture, gait, and activities. In addition to monitoring normal daily activities and detecting potential adverse events such as falls, the UbiSense system aims to capture signs of deterioration of the patients by analyzing subtle changes in posture and gait. One of the major challenges of vision-based systems is the perceived intrusion of privacy because of the way that image data are transmitted and analyzed. To circumvent this problem, the captured images in UbiSense are immediately filtered at the device level into blobs, which encapsulate only the shape outline and motion vectors of the subject. Visual images are not stored or transmitted at any stage of the process so that it is impossible to reconstruct the abstract information back into the original image. The posture is estimated by fusing multiple cues obtained from the blobs and comparing them with reference patterns of the common postures. From the posture estimation results, activity can be accurately determined. For example, if the resident falls on the floor while attempting to get out of a chair, the posture is expected to change from sitting to standing to finally lying down. If the posture analysis algorithm detects an activity characterized by such a posture change pattern, the system can be set to raise a fall alarm. Experimental results on a simulated dataset show an average accuracy of 90% in identifying different postures.

Another video processing-based fall detection system, being developed at the University of Dundee, uses ceiling-mounted visual sensors to monitor a supportive home environment [36]. Ceiling-mounted sensors are preferred over the wall-mounted sensors as they minimize occlusion of the person by furniture. Standard cameras, as opposed to infra-red, are employed in this study as they are relatively cheaper. Patterns of inactivity could be used to make inferences about health and also to help detect falls. However, the significance of inactivity changes with context. A person lying on a sofa, as one often does, is probably only resting. In contrast, a person lying on the floor, where one is not expected to lay, may have fallen and require assistance. This monitoring system uses the information of contextual inactivity to detect falls when extended localization of a person is observed outside the normal inactivity zones. This information when combined with information about body pose and motion provides a useful cue for fall detection. The sensitivity or specificity of this system has not been evaluated.

The Smart Inactivity Monitor Using Array-Based Detectors (SIMBAD) fall detector, developed at the University of Liverpool, uses a low-cost array of infrared detectors to capture low-level image of the resident and then analyzes the subject's motion to detect a fall event [37]. The IRISYS sensors used in this detector tracks the moving objects and provides a way of non-intrusive monitoring because of the low resolution of the captured images. The information of the size, location, and velocity of the moving object is determined using image-processing algorithms. Falls are detected based on the velocity and acceleration of the tracked object. In this study, neural networks were used to classify falls. The performance of the SIMBAD fall detector was tested by emulating different types of fall (for example, slipping and tripping) with varied movement dynamics, viewpoints, and degrees of obscuration in a controlled laboratory set up. Although the system exhibited good specificity in terms of low false-alarm rates, it could detect only 30% of the emulated falls. The authors attributed the poor performance to inadequate training set, and a better performance was projected on using generalized training sets that are sufficiently varied and viewpoint invariant.

Generally, all the video-based fall-monitoring systems have the potential to automatically detect falls with no user intervention and also overcome the problem of stigmatization to an extent, as they do not require the users to wear any devices. However, the fear of intrusion of privacy is more prominent in the camera-centric technologies. Despite using a low-quality imaging and/or on-site image processing, the residents may still experience the feeling of "being-watched" based on their perceptions of the sensor. The devices in this category also generally have higher cost than automatic wearable fall detectors, because of the need for more intensive computations.

Floor Vibration-Based Fall Detectors

There are also two classes of vibration-based systems. The first uses acoustic analysis of the sounds made by the body when it falls. For floor surfaces such as wooden boards, the sounds of an impact are very distinctive and can easily be distinguished from dropped items such as a tray or a book. However, acoustic analysis is very difficult in the case of common floors such as concrete covered with rugs or carpets [33]. The second approach involves a direct conversion of mechanical energy associated with the impact on the floor into an electrical signal using vibration sensors. One of recent fall detectors that fall in this category is a fall detector that is being developed in the Medical Automation Research Center (MARC) at the University of Virginia [38–40]. The design and the working principle of this detector are explained in some detail in what follows.

The working of the floor vibration-based fall detector is founded on the hypothesis that it is possible *to detect human falls by observing the vibration patterns in the floor*.

The above hypothesis, essentially, implies that (i) the vibration signature of the floor generated by a fall is significantly different from those generated by normal daily activities such as walking, tapping, etc. and (ii) the vibration signature of the floor generated by a human fall is significantly different from those generated by falling objects.

The floor vibration-based fall detector, shown in Fig. 8.5, uses a special piezoelectric sensor coupled to the floor surface by means of mass and spring arrangement, combined with preprocessing electronics to evaluate the vibrations of the floor. The whole detector set up weighs around 3.5 pounds and can be placed directly on the floor, typically one per large room. The detector continuously monitors the floor for vibrations that are produced by the common activities of the resident such as walking, sitting down, tapping, etc.

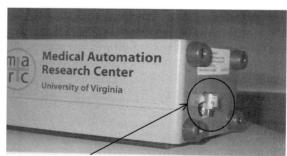

Fig. 8.5 Floor
Vibration-based Fall Detector   Piezo Transducer

On the basis of the experiments conducted, it was noted that there were significant differences in the patterns of vibrations induced on the floor by different activities. There was also a significant difference in the vibration pattern generated by a falling object as opposed to those generated by a falling anthropomorphic dummy, which in this case is representative of a human fall. This difference in floor response for different activities was effectively exploited to detect the falls with a higher degree of sensitivity and fewer false positives. The device detects a fall only when the vibration pattern (frequency, amplitude, duration, etc.) obtained from the floor over a small period of time matches the pattern induced when a person falls on the floor. The detector can then report the fall alert to the responder through an appropriate communications portal such as utilizing the telephone to send a message to a radio pager or to a cellular phone. Figure 8.6 depicts a schematic representation of the various stages that the fall detector goes through to report the fall to the responder following the event of a resident fall.

The performance of the detector was evaluated by conducting controlled laboratory trials. Human falls were simulated using anthropomorphic dummies, which have mass distribution similar to those of humans and hence can give a good representation of a human fall's effect on the floor. The fall tests were conducted on mezzanine concrete floor and concrete slab floors. A Hybrid-III seated crash test dummy, weighing 180 pounds, and a Rescue Randy, a 6-foot, 1-inch tall dummy weighing 165 pounds were used in the tests. The Hybrid-III dummy was used to emulate the scenario of a person falling when attempting to get out from a chair/wheelchair and the Rescue Randy was used to emulate tripping and falling from an upright position.

The ability of the fall detector to distinguish a human fall from an object dropped within the detection range was evaluated by dropping objects weighing 5 and 15 pounds, representative of weights of common objects in a residential set up, at various distances covering the entire range of fall detection up to 20 feet. Figure 8.7 shows the vibration signal of the floor, as measured by the piezoelectric sensor, for a Rescue Randy fall at a distance of 20 feet. This vibration pattern is significantly different from the one that is produced by an object fall as close as 2 feet from the sensor, shown in Fig. 8.8.

On the basis of the tests conducted, the fall detection range for the sensor was found to be 20 feet in the case of mezzanine concrete floor covered with linoleum and 15 feet on concrete slab floor. It was observed that the fall detector circuitry required different processing thresholds depending on the dynamic properties of

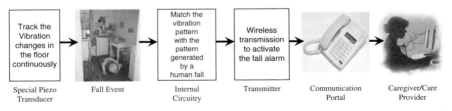

Fig. 8.6 Schematic Representation of the Working Principle of the Floor Vibration-Based Fall Detector

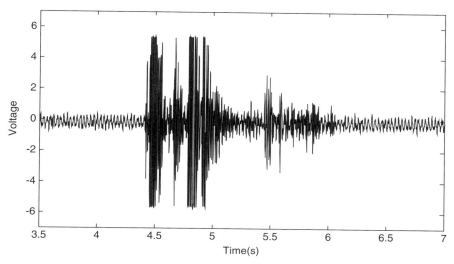

Fig. 8.7 Pre-amplified signal from the piezoelectric sensor showing the vibration pattern of the floor following the event of a Rescue Randy fall, at a distance of 20 feet from the sensor, on Mezzanine concrete floor covered with linoleum

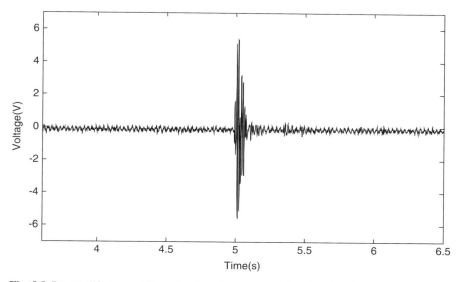

Fig. 8.8 Pre-amplified signal from the piezoelectric sensor showing the vibration pattern of the floor following a 15 lb object fall, at a distance of 2 feet from the sensor, on Mezzanine concrete floor covered with linoleum

the floor. This can be achieved by means of a simple toggle switch that selects threshold levels and sensitivities appropriate to the floor type where the device is installed. Utilizing these modifications in settings, the fall detection function produced impressive repeatable performance on both mezzanine concrete and concrete slab floors. Controlled experiments conducted to test this fall detector attained 100% true positives and 0% false alarms, which is clearly much better than most of the other types of fall detectors. Besides being passive (as the user is not required to wear any device), the detector is also unobtrusive as compared with the video monitoring-based fall detectors. This device is currently undergoing testing in real-life setting.

8.3 Conclusion

Technology may be used to reduce the burden of falls at several stages of prevention by alerting caregivers to intervene and prevent a fall, limiting morbidity from a fall by reducing the impact to the faller, and by reducing response time for rescue or intervention. Advances in material sciences and future developments may lead to economic passive prevention technologies such as better floors for frail elders to live on, which provide all the stability of a firm surface, but provide absorption of enough energy to prevent harm to the faller, and possibly integrate sensor technologies for the detection of falls.

References

1. Centers for Disease Control and Prevention. Web-based Injury Statistics Query and Reporting System (WISQARS) [Online]. (2005). National Center for Injury Prevention and Control, Centers for Disease Control and Prevention (producer). Available from: URL: www.cdc.gov/ncipc/wisqars.
2. Sterling DA, O'Connor JA, Bonadies J. Geriatric falls: injury severity is high and disproportionate to mechanism. Journal of Trauma-Injury Infection and Critical Care 2001, 50(1):116–9.
3. Rizzo JA, et al. Health care utilization and costs in a Medicare population by fall status. Medical Care 1998, 36(8):1174–88.
4. Cumming RG, Kelsey JL, Nevitt MC. Methodologic issues in the study of frequent and recurrent health problems. Falls in the elderly. Ann Epidemiology. 1990, 1:49–56.
5. Stevens JA, et al. The costs of fatal and nonfatal falls among older adults. Injury Prevention 2006, 12:290–5.
6. Magaziner J, et al. Recovery from hip fracture in eight areas of function. Journal of Gerontology: Medical Sciences 2000, 55A(9):M498–507.
7. Guideline for the Prevention of Falls in Older Persons. JAGS 2001; 49:664–672. (same as #17 American Geriatrics Society, British Geriatrics Society, and American Academy of Orthopaedic Surgeons Panel on Falls Prevention, "Guideline for the prevention of falls in older persons", Journal of the American Geriatric Society. 2001, 49:664–672.)
8. Gryfe CI, Amies A, Ashley MJ. "A Longitudinal Study of Falls in an Elderly Population: I. Incidence and Morbidity", Age Ageing, 1977.

9. Jensen J, et al. Falls among frail older people in residential care. Scand J Public Health 2002, 30:54–61.
10. Beauchet O, et al. "Factors contributing to falls in elderly subjects leading to acute-care hospitalization", La Presse Medicale, 29(28):1544–1548, 2000.
11. Ugur C., et al. "Characteristics of falling in patients with stroke", Journal of Neurology, Neurosurgery, and Psychiatry, 69(5):649–651, 2000.
12. Lipsitz, AL, et al. "Causes and correlates of recurrent falls in ambulatory in frail elderly." Journal of Gerontology: Medical Sciences, 46(4):114–122.
13. Leipzig MR, et al. "Drugs and falls in older people: a systematic review and meta-analysis: I. psychotropic drugs." Journal of American Geriatric Society, 47(1):30–39, 1999.
14. Kiely KD, et al. "Identifying nursing home residents at risk for falling", Journal of the American Geriatric Society, 46(5):551–555, 1998.
15. Tinetti, Mary E. MD. Preventing Falls in Elderly Persons. NEJM 2003; 348(1):42–49.
16. Oliver D, et al. Strategies to prevent falls and fractures in hospitals and care homes and effect of cognitive impairment: systematic review and meta-analyses BMJ. 334(7584):82, 2007.
17. Chang, John T. Interventions for the prevention of falls in older adults: systematic review and meta-analysis of randomized clinical trials. BMJ 2004: 328; 610–617.
18. Morse, J, et al. "Development of a scale to identify the fall-prone patient," Canadian Journal on Ageing, 8(4):366–377, 1989.
19. Heslin K, et al. "Managing falls: Identifying population specific risk factors and prevention strategies." In S. Funk, E. Tornquist, M. Champagne & R. Weise (Eds.). "Key Aspects of Elder Care: Managing Falls, Incontinence, and Cognitive Impairment" (pp 70–88), New York: Springer Publishing, 1992.
20. Tinetti TL, Liu W, Ginter S. "Mechanical restraint use and fall-related injuries among residents of skilled nursing facilities," Annuals of Internal Medicine, 116:369–374, 1992.
21. Evans L, et al. "A clinical trial to reduce restraints in nursing homes." Journal of the American Geriatrics Society, 45:675–81, 1997.
22. Ash LK, Macleod P, Clark L. "A case control study of falls in the hospital setting." Journal of Gerontological Nursing, 24(12):7–15, 1998.
23. Nakamura D, Holm M, Wilson A. "Measures of balance and fear of falling in the elderly: A review." Physical and Occupational Therapy in Geriatrics, 15(4):17–32, 1998.
24. Tideiksaar R, Feiner CF, Maby J. "Falls prevention: The efficacy of a bed alarm system in an acute-care setting." Mt Sinai J Med 1993;60:522–527.
25. Mayo NE, Gloutney L, Levy AR. "A randomized trial of identification bracelets to prevent falls among patients in a rehabilitation hospital." Arch Phys Med Rehabil 1994, 74:1302–1308.
26. Kelly, et al. "Evaluation of a Nonintrusive Monitor to Reduce Falls in Nursing Home Patients." J Am Med Dir Assoc 2002, 3:377–382.
27. Kannus P, et al. "Prevention of hip fracture in elderly people with use of a hip protector." N Engl J Med 2000, 343:1506–1513.
28. Parker MJ, Gillespie WJ, Gillespie LD. Effectiveness of hip protectors for preventing hip fractures in elderly people: systematic review. BMJ. 332(7541):571–4, 2006.
29. Sawka AM, et al.. Do hip protectors decrease the risk of hip fracture in institutional and community-dwelling elderly? A systematic review and meta-analysis of randomized controlled trials Osteoporosis International. 16(12):1461–74, 2005.
30. Casalena JA, et al. 1998. The Penn State Safety Floor: Part I–Design Parameters Associated with Walking Deflections. Journal of Biomechanical Engineering. 120:518–526.
31. Casalena JA, et al. 1998. The Penn State Safety Floor: Part II–Reduction of Fall-Related Peak Impact Forces on the Femur. Journal of Biomechanical Engineering. 120:527–532.
32. Doughty K, "Fall Prevention and Management Strategies Based on Intelligent Detection, Monitoring and Assessment." Presented at "New Technologies in Medicine for the Elderly", Charing Cross Hospital, 30th. Nov. 2000.
33. Hwang JY, et al. "Development of Novel Algorithm and Real-time Monitoring Ambulatory System Using Bluetooth Module for Fall Detection in the Elderly." Proceedings of the 26th Annual International Conference of the IEEE EMBS, 2004.

34. Degen T, et al. "Speedy: A fall detector in a wristwatch," 7th International Symposium on Wearable Computers (ISWC), White Plains, NY, Oct. 2003, pp. 184–189.

35. Benny PL, et al. "From imaging networks to behavior profiling: ubiquitous sensing for managed homecare of the elderly." Adjunct Proceedings of the 3rd International Conference on Pervasive Computing (PERVASIVE 2005), pp. 101–104, May 2005.

36. Nait CH, McKenna SJ. "Activity summarisation and fall detection in a supportive home environment", Int. Conf. on Pattern Recognition (ICPR), 2004.

37. Sixsmith A, Johnson N. "Smart sensor to detect the falls of the elderly", IEEE Pervasive Computing, vol. 3, no. 2, pp. 42–47, April-June 2004.

38. Alwan M, et al. "Derivation of Basic Human Gait Characteristics from Floor Vibrations", 2003 Summer Bioengineering Conference, June 25–29, Key Biscayne FL.

39. Rajendran P, et al. "A Passive Floor-Vibration Based Fall Detector", 2006 International Conf on Aging, Disability and Independence, Feb 1–4, St.Petersburg FL.

40. Alwan M, et al. "A Smart and Passive Floor-Vibration Based Fall Detector for Elderly", 2nd IEEE International Conference on Information and Communication Technologies, 2006.

Chapter 9
Computerized Methods for Cognitive Testing

Vered Aharonson and Amos D. Korczyn

9.1 The Scope of the Problem

Most authorities consider Alzheimer disease (AD) to be the most common type of dementia in people above age 70, and accumulating evidence shows that the prevalence of the disease is on the increase and will reach pandemic proportions with the aging of the population. While the underlying processes are being explored, several risk factors have already been identified, which can delineate those at higher risk (Table 9.1). In parallel, a huge effort is being made to find interventions that will cure AD or at least stop its progression. Once successful, these methods could only be useful if AD is diagnosed early, either presymptomatically or in the stage now termed mild cognitive impairment (MCI) [1].

However, not all elderly people who have cognitive impairment necessarily have AD as the underlying pathology. There are a large number of other causes for cognitive decline (Table 9.2), many of which are treatable. These disorders should also be identified at an early stage to allow proper treatment.

Over the years, several methods have been used to diagnose dementia at an early stage. Most of those use AD as the template disorder. While this approach has advantages, missing cases with non-AD pathologies should be minimized.

Moreover, not all elderly people who feel that their cognitive function has deteriorated actually have incipient dementia. It is also very important to identify, diagnose, and give proper advice to those cases who are "worried well."

Thus, it seems that an attempt should be made to screen elderly people for cognitive impairment. This can be done through a multi-level approach, starting with those who themselves complain of impairment, or at least acknowledge its existence, then those who are at particular risk (positive family history or other genetic risk factors, or any of the other risk factors mentioned in Table 9.1), and later all others.

The mere number of such candidates excludes most of the screening methods that are listed in Table 9.3, which are either prohibitively expensive, too long to

Vered Aharonson
Department of Software Engineering, Tel Aviv Academic College of Engineering, Afeka, Israel
e-mail: vered@afeka.ac.il

From: *Aging Medicine, Eldercare Technology for Clinical Practitioners,*
Edited by: M. Alwan and R. Felder © Humana Press, Totowa, NJ

Table 9.1 Risk factors for dementia

Age
Female sex
Head trauma
Low level of education
Smoking
Diabetes mellitus
Hypertension
Apolipoprotein E e 4
Coronary artery disease
High dietary saturated fat and cholesterol
Hyperhomocysteinemia
Depression

Table 9.2 Most common causes of dementia

Alzheimer's disease
Vascular dementia
Lewy body dementia
Frontotemporal dementia

Table 9.3 Dementia screening methods

Structural/Functional MRI
Brain metabolism/amyloid imaging
Neuropsychological tests

perform, and/or demand an expert to administer them (a physician, neuropsychologist, radiologist, etc.). Computerized assessment can be considered as alternative to those processes or at least the initial screening phase of the process of cognitive evaluation, before other methods of evaluation will be employed.

9.2 Usefulness of Computerized Testing

During the last two decades, there has been a rush to computerize tasks of our daily life, personal and professional. Computers offer the potential to make things easier, more affordable, or more efficient. Each new application claims to provide additional benefits. In some cases and for some users, however, the latter claim does not hold, and the computerization not only fails to facilitate the execution of a task but even unfortunately worsens it.

To understand the reason for this phenomenon, the field of usability offers two measures: usability and usefulness [2]. The two are often mixed and, indeed, in some cases are related, but in fact they are very distinct entities.

Usefulness can be defined as an improvement of a certain process without decreasing its previous advantages and benefits. For example, writing a book chapter using a computer's text editor is an improvement to the previous method, the typing machine. The texts can still be typed using the same practice on the keyboard, but corrections are easier to do and "cut and paste", and spelling options have been added. In addition, the files are easier to handle; they can be electronically stored, retrieved, printed, and sent by email to co-writers. In comparison, reading a book from a computer screen is disadvantageous to be a good replacement to the old-fashioned paper book. Reading from the screen is fatiguing to the eyes; the screen in often not big enough to accommodate a whole page and scrolling back and forth is needed. The simple task of flipping to the next page also becomes annoying, using keyboard keys or the computer mouse. And above all, one does not have the "feel" of sitting comfortably on an armchair, opening a book, and feeling the touch and smell of paper.

Usability assesses the manner in which a system has been designed. Bad design can result in a sorely disappointing experience to the user and can make a potentially useful technology unusable in practice. Usability will be discussed in the next section.

Cognitive testing is a very intricate task, which involves many issues, from medical to social, legal, and cultural. One must consider carefully whether a computerized version of those tests is useful or advantageous.

We will now proceed to look at the usefulness of cognitive testing performed by a computer.

9.2.1 The Advantages and Limitations of Pen-and-Paper Tests

To evaluate the usefulness of computerized cognitive testing, we shall consider first the inherent features of traditional methods that are currently used to perform cognitive tests.

Traditionally, most cognitive tests are pen-and-paper forms or oral questionnaires that are administered by a professional person. This person provides explanation on how to fill the forms or to perform the tasks involved and observes the subjects as they go through the tasks. The administrator should be skillful to interpret correctly the subject's reactions to the explanations given to determine whether the subject had understood the task and is ready to start the test. Administrators also monitor their subjects during the test to help them avoid or overcome difficulties. There are two inherent disadvantages in this process. One is that a professional person is needed to administer tests and questionnaires that are sometimes simple and straightforward to subjects who often do not need explanations or monitoring. The professional person can, in those cases, make better use of the time dealing with more intricate cases of diagnosis and treatment. More importantly, the process is not standardized. Different administrators give different explanations, in different length or different intonations. In such cases, some subjects may get more help when taking the test than others. The mood of an administrator can vary from one day to another, causing his/her to treat different subjects differently. The latter point can be an upside, as different subjects may need different attitudes. However, a human administrator cannot record quantitatively the help given to each subject. How can one describe a "manner of speech" or "pace of delivering instructions"? Even if those attributes are described and written in a session's summary, the resulting document will be very subjective and non-standard. A more difficult question is how to consider such "modifications of attitude" in the interpretation of the subject's performance.

If differences in the administration process are not taken into account in the scoring paradigm, the scores may become non-standard and biased. Pen-and-paper tests are scored manually. This process is both tedious and prone to errors. Sometimes the scores are delayed for several days before they can be handed or sent to the referring doctor or the subject.

Another practical issue is the storage and retrieval of test results. The test scores need to be stored and filed. It takes time to search for a form every time it is required for discussion or healthcare professionals' consultations. A form needs to be copied and either faxed or put in an envelope and send by post to distant health professionals or to the subject.

Excellent cognitive tests have been developed and used over the last 50 years. Different tests evaluate different cognitive domains at different levels, and there is a problem as to which test should be used. The administrator, in such cases, has to go through many forms and decide on the spot which ones to use. This process is not only inefficient but also non-uniform, as not all subjects will get identical tests in a given situation.

The above mentioned tests have been validated in careful research as good measures for the cognitive functions they explore. Those measures, however, depend on norms that have been determined back then. As those norms date back several decades, they need to be undated and re-established. This process is costly and labor intensive.

9.2.2 The Trouble with Computers

Computers can help to overcome many of the abovementioned limitations. They can efficiently store any amount of data and make it easy to retrieve and transmit. A computer administers the cognitive test in exactly the same manner every time and this makes it objective and standard. If tasks and/or their explanations are altered in a computerized cognitive testing session, this fact can be recorded and stored with the test results and may be used in the interpretation process. Score calculation is automatic and immediate. Tests can be dynamically chosen from a large arsenal of options to accommodate different subjects and different cognitive levels. New norms can be periodically and automatically calculated if controls data are accumulated in a central database.

Computers, however, have their own drawbacks. One inherent reason for this is that a wide range of things performed by humans cannot be taken over completely by machines. People can persuade, socialize, understand feelings, reach decisions, etc. None of these has yet been or is likely to be soon implemented in computers. A computer system can be useful, however, in specific tasks or parts of a task so that they can act as assistants or "power tools."

People are often reluctant to use computerized cognitive tests and claim that they are not useful due to the fact that a computer, like any technology, requires a change of a process. This claim is in part emotional, the natural aversion to "break up with the past," but objective usefulness problems exist as well. A computer that administers cognitive tests need to be bought. It needs to be placed on a designated table, sometimes in a designated room. Often it needs to be connected to the Internet to transmit the test for analysis. All these increase the cost of installation. The staff of a clinic needs to be trained to use the new technology and those people often raise resistance because of their instinctive fear that their jobs will be hampered and that "the computer may eventually substitute them."

Subjects who need to take computerized cognitive tests have their own apprehensions and anxieties concerning the technology. Very often they need extra convincing and encouragement to even start tasks involving computer usage. Thus, a computerized process that could be, in principle, shorter and more efficient often becomes complicated and cumbersome.

9.3 Usability of Computerized Testing

Many of the "troubles with computers" mentioned in the previous section stem from bad design that do not follow the usability requirements. An inadequate or erroneous design can make both test administrators and examinees experience an unpleasant and frustrating inadequacy when activating and using the computerized tests. If a system is designed in a way that is understandable to the user and can be quickly learned and implemented, the reluctance to use it can be overcome. Allan Cooper from Mackintosh, in his book *The Inmates are Running the Asylum* [3], calls this phenomenon "Software Apartheid," where talented and intelligent people are forbidden from doing a job because they cannot use computers effectively. There are plenty of methods in which software can be designed to be more "human" and "forgiving," thus becoming accommodating.

The inadequacy issue is particularly important when the technology is targeted to elderly people. Young people were born to the digital age. They are skillful with computers and tolerate easily their "bad behavior." People in their 40s or 50s who were exposed to computers in their 20s or 30s sometimes have experience with computers. It is the elderly who find those computers frightening and are flustered and bewildered by them. In cognitive testing for the elderly, a majority of the target users might experience those negative reactions. This fact must be taken carefully into account as this can eliminate all the advantages and reproduce the limitation of human administration.

9.3.1 Optimal Length of a Computerized Battery

Oral or pen-and-paper tests can sometime take a long time to administer. A skillful and experienced administrator can sense when the subject gets too tired to go on or suddenly loses concentration and give the subject a break, send the subject to drink water or rest, before resuming the testing session. In a computerized examination, fatigue may set in much earlier; even a good computer screen is fatiguing to the eyes. Handling a computer mouse is tiring to the hand and arm, especially to those inexperienced in computer usage. Usability tests have shown that even young people sense a considerable decline in concentration after 40 min of working with a computer. Elderly people feel this in a stronger way. A cognitive test battery should be therefore limited to 40 min at most.

9.3.2 Computer Experience

Most elderly people have no computer skills or computer experience. They are reluctant to take a computerized test, and when persuaded to take it, they feel anxious and bewildered. This fact can severely hinge the performance of those subjects and lead to erroneous test results. One solution to this problem is to have only computer-skilled people take the computerized test, but this cannot offer standardization to the cognitive evaluation of an elderly population. A good design of computerized testing should minimize the anxiety of such persons and adjust the computer interaction required to their capabilities. For example, the computer should be sensitive to hesitations, slow reaction, or missing reactions from the user and provide help. The user should feel that the computer is differential to him or her and that the computer is forthcoming with information about what he or she has to do next. The computer should anticipate its user's needs and respond to them. In short, instead of being an interface, the software should interact with the users. The design should be based on human behavior and consider what is valuable to the user in the first place.

9.3.3 Motor Skills

Typing on a computer keyboard and using the computer mouse may be difficult for elderly people who have motor problems but can also be challenging to normal elderly who have not previously been trained with those specific motor functions. Computer mouse operations in particular are usually not feasible for elderly people over 85. One advantage of computer testing is the ability to measure accurately reaction time. However, in the case of lack of motor skills, those reaction time measurements mean very little and even worse, they bias the interpretation of the performance. There should be an adaptive process in the computer's hardware and software that detects and estimates the effect of insufficient motor skills and takes them into account. This process should be implemented in the administration of those tests, giving persons with motor problems more time to react. Motor skills should also be taken into account in the interpretation of the users' performance. Slowness because of cognitive decline should be distinguished from motor disorders or difficulties' effects.

9.3.4 Education

The problem of limited or no education is often related to the lack of computer experience but can also be manifested independently. The language issue is important for people with low education. Instructions should be simple using easy wording and sometimes repeated several times. Human administrators usually do this instinctively. However, this "instinctive" adjustment to only some subjects, without an ability to quantify and record the change in instruction complexity, hampers standardability and objectivity. Software can implement a vast arsenal of instruction options, in different complexity levels, and use them discriminately for different users while recording the instruction set used. This mechanism should also encompass an interpretation method that will be able to evaluate the performance of the users in conjugation with the level of the instruction given to them.

People who cannot read and write should have an alternative to written instructions. A voice interface is useful for these individuals. Recorded instructions can easily be used. However, speech recognition technology is not yet ripe to understand a user's voiced answers. Current speech recognition technologies still suffer from high error rate, especially in spontaneous speech recognition, thus making existing speech recognition engines un-usable for those types of applications. Speech technology, however, is advancing at steady pace, and in several years time those limitations might be removed.

9.3.5 Domains Tested

Almost all pen-and-paper tests can in principle be translated to computerized versions. However, some cognitive domains tested by oral tests are difficult to implement. Therefore, verbal skills cannot be communicated to the "testing computer" by typing and should be administered by a voice interface. Many tasks that are related to executive functions need drawing on paper and those are difficult to implement with the computer mouse. Even very skilled people find it hard to draw using a computer mouse. The design of tests for those cognitive domains should include usable accessories and technology attached to them that will enable to perform verbal and intricate motor tasks.

9.3.6 Software Versus Hardware

Some computerized tests today try to overcome usability problems by employing specialized hardware. For example, some systems use touch screens instead of a keyboard. This poses a new set of difficulties. One is the expense attached to purchasing such a hardware. The normal PC has become a commodity and its prices are dropping. On the other hand, a small clinic or one that performs limited number of cognitive tests will find it problematic to start using a system that needs touch screen.

Moreover, experience has shown that even with touch screens, there are usability problems. If the explanation and examples are not clear enough and the system is not responsive enough to the subject's difficulties and needs, the expensive hardware is not of much help. Using a touch screen for long periods may cause physical burden for elderly subjects as it involves continuous pointing with the whole arm on the screen, as opposed to placing the hands on a desktop keyboard, which is a natural movement.

9.3.7 Sub-Tests and Task Variations

An important advantage of computerized administration is that the computer can efficiently choose from a large arsenal of tests, the ones to include in each testing session. A test is usually composed of a sequence of tasks that the subject has to fulfill. The order of the tasks as well as their contents can also be easily varied in computer test administration. The latter feature is very important in the case of re-test; if the tasks are varied in a follow-up session, the subject cannot "prepare" or "learn" tests or tasks that were administered to him or her previously and thus can, in principle, take a test as often as needed. The problem is a naïve design of choosing a test that randomly lacks the expertise of a human administrator who adjusts the task to the subject's performance. Although difficult to implement, an automated adjustment mechanism should be used in the digital form of those tests. The complexity of the task, the time given to complete them, and the instructions attached to them should be adaptive and follow closely the user's performance.

9.3.8 Data Handling—Security Issues

Handling a paper test form may be cumbersome, but its safety can be easily accomplished. A paper form can be locked in a cupboard in secured clinic building, and can be accessed by authorized personnel only, who can then provide the information to designated people. When using digital data, especially in computers connected to the Internet, the safety and privacy issues must be very carefully considered. The protocols involved in the medical data handling and transmission should be followed closely.

9.4 Validation of New Techniques

A new issue that emerges from the proliferation of computerized cognitive testing is the need for a paradigm of validation that will be required for their acceptance in clinical or other settings. A vast knowledge has accumulated in industry nowadays about quality assessment practices for technologies. One of the keywords in this field is benchmarks. A benchmark is a point of reference against which something may be compared. Industry defines those references where every new solution can be tested, and its results compared to other solutions. Often a technology needs to be tested on a set of benchmarks. The characteristics of each benchmark are carefully defined for each technology [4].

The definition of "benchmark" in the field of computerized cognitive evaluation is, however, tricky compared to other "detection" technologies. For example, technologies of speech recognition are tested on a group of recorded speech, where the number of correctly recognized words can be compared. Compression technologies are tested on a group of documents, where the resulting size of the documents is compared.

Cognitive testing is done on humans. Naturally, one cannot have the same group of people available to all computerized batteries, and even if that could be managed, the dynamic nature of human behavior will make intrinsic differences not related to the technologies themselves. For example, the order in which the different tests are presented to the subjects will influence the subject's performance. However, one can define a "profile" of a test population that would be a standard testing ground for different technologies. Such a profile can be described as a matrix of age groups, education levels, computer skills, and motor skills.

Cognitive testing technologies, computerized or not, have exclusion criteria or the type of subjects who cannot use it. It stands to reason that paralyzed, blind, or deaf persons might be excluded from some programs. There are programs limited to certain language or languages and therefore exclude all people who do not speak those languages. However, one should be careful not to exclude too many subjects! If certain cognitive test is limited to persons below the age of 40, naturally it cannot be applied to elderly for the detection of dementia.

Once a "benchmark population" has been established, a methodology and measures should be depicted to evaluate the technology's performance. For computerized cognitive assessment, the validity of its results and its reliability in terms of test–retest should be examined. The latter task is the easier of the two. The "benchmark" subjects can have a baseline examination using the technology and then retested after an agreed elapsed time.

The validity measures are much more complex to define as they entail a comparison to a "gold standard." If the tests that were computerized are known traditional neuropsychological tests that have been validated, the process is relatively straight forward; the computerized tests' outcome can be compared to the traditional methods' outcome. Manual neuropsychological tests are lengthy and each tests a specific cognitive domain so that a large set of such tests is required. The procedure thence becomes long and costly.

Some software, however, use novel neuropsychological tests that have not been previously validated. Those are more difficult to evaluate, as the effect of computerization on the evaluation is hard to assess. One solution is to use the best "gold standard," for example, a professional expert, either physician or neuropsychologist. Often, however, experts differ in their evaluations. A good practice would then be to have three specialists examine each subject and stipulate a "majority vote" for the resulting diagnosis. This, of course, is a costly method. Another method often used is a comparison to manual screening tests, like the Mini Mental State Examination (MMSE). Although the MMSE has been around for many years and has become a sort of standard, health professionals agree that it is very coarse in its cognitive evaluation performance. It can and indeed is being used, however, as a screening tool for subjects' recruitment for clinical trials and therefore can be used as a part of the benchmark definition.

It should be emphasized that the difficulties mentioned stem from the novelty of the field of computerized tests. We are indeed in a beginning of an era, when computerized cognitive testing has just begun its penetration. Once validation standards are chosen and established and existing technologies tested, the relevant medical associations can determine based on the performance results a "winning" solution that will be made a "new standard for computerized cognitive tests" and serve as comparison tool to validation of new technologies that will emerge.

9.5 Existing approaches

The need for computerized cognitive assessments technology yielded several commercial companies who now offer a variety of solutions. As a comprehensive, standard validation paradigm is not yet established, when comparing different solutions, one has to consider the characteristics of each and discuss their advantages in terms of usability by elderly and health professionals attending to them.

The first issue to consider is the target application of the technology and whether the solution provided is designed for elderly care application. It turns out that several solutions were designed and intended for clinical trials. There is little doubt that computerization can enhance and facilitate the search for drugs and treatments for AD and other cognitive diseases and disorders. However, both needs and facilities in the research environment are very different from those in health care settings. Solutions for research settings are characterized by a multitude of attractive computerized tests that could fit a variety of research goals. Available solutions include CDR®, CANTAB®, and COGTEST®. The first two were the first in the market and were successful to meet the needs of various studies since. Research is, however, characterized by dedicated personnel, who can spend as much time as needed to administer the computerized assessments, inform and instruct the subjects tested, and basically, cover any usability weaknesses of the computerized solution. The computer in those applications yields a more or less standardized testing session and handles efficiently the results storage for analysis. This scenario is very difficult to imitate in a healthcare setting, where the personnel is fully occupied with attending the patients, and extra help for administering the computer assessment is rarely available. Solutions specifically designed for applications of healthcare are Mindstreams® and NexAde®.

Another consideration is the target population of the solution. It is business-wise logical to have as larger a scope as possible for a solution. However, it is evident that usability-wise, a solution cannot fit ages "nine to ninety." Using computerized tests to assess cognitive state of children versus young people versus people over 65 necessitates more than just different tasks and questionnaires. A specific computer usability platform should be designed and tested to fit each target population. The same goes for cognitive assessment in different diseases. Computerized cognitive assessments aimed at Parkinson's disease subjects or people with head injuries need different considerations in the solution design. A solution that conforms to being limited to the elderly population (60+), to dementia screening, and to healthcare settings is the NexAde® [5, 6].

Some solutions (CANTAB®, IntegNeuro®, and CANS-MCI®) use non-standard accessories, namely touch screens to ease the computer interaction for the subject. CANS-MCI® provides an alternative to the touch screen in the form of a computer mouse, but there again, this interface is unusable for elderly. Touch screens indeed facilitate the user's interaction with the computer as "pointing at a screen" is a natural gesture. However, even those costly accessories often do not solve the usability problem. There are many "interface layers" that contribute to the experience of the user and should be considered when trying to facilitate the human–computer interaction. Those interface layers include instructions, explanations, examples and training, and coherent feedback to the subject's actions. The layers should also be adjusted to the subject's performance abilities. A non-adjusted interface layer can cause frustration to the "weak" user or be irritating to a "strong" one. An interesting solution was proposed and implemented by NexAde® [7]. The interface is adjusted to the subjects by use of a "user profile" that is calculated throughout this computerized assessment, and a timely adjustment of the interface is initiated by the software.

Many solutions include an impressive collection of tests that encompass a wide range of cognitive functions. As stated before, it is very important to limit the length of the computerized testing session to a maximum of 40 min that will not compromise the attention of the subject. Although several existing solutions state that they take "approximately 30 min" (CDR®) or "20–40 min" (NeuroTrax®), they actually take longer when employed by elderly who have cognitive impairment and/or are computer naïve, with no administrator to handle part of the computer operations. Those latter subjects are the ones whose fatigue will set even earlier than cognitively intact, computer-skilled subjects and might bias their performance analysis. Those fatigue phenomena might be detected and dealt with by a human administrator sitting with the subject by the computer, but this triggers other complications, as was discussed before, by making the assessment non-standard. Moreover, some subjects tire even before 40 min have elapsed. As always with usability, there is no "magic number" giving an optimal test length for all subjects. One solution is to adjust the assessment's length according to the subject's performance, using the detection of decline in attention as a precursor to an abort of the program [8].

As mentioned before, the need for humans to administer the computerized tests sitting with the subjects by a computer is not a good solution neither practically and budget-wise nor clinically, because of administrator's bias. Several solutions (CogHealth®, NeuroTrax®, CANS-MCI®, and NexAde®) claim to be suitable for self-administration. It is hard to assess the validity of those statements, as they stem from experimental settings and not "real-world" clinical ones. Those claims will have to be validated using a standard benchmark.

9.6 Needs and Future Development

We are at the beginning of an era of computerization for cognitive and behavioral testing tools. The vision of this field is to have computers simulate to a better extent the "human touch" while still preserving the advantages of computers—accuracy, objectivity, and data-handling capabilities (like storage and transmission). Progress is made daily toward this goal. Computers now come with "eyes and ears," standard and cheap accessories like video-cam and microphone, which can capture the user's facial expressions and voice. The "brains" of the machine, its algorithms and software, are also developing; signal processing tools now enable more accurate detection and selection of characteristics of human expression (speech and movements). Non-deterministic decision tools like neural networks enable more flexible handling of the data derived by the signal processing modules.

Of course, it is intuitively as well as mathematically [9] obvious that computers will never have full human capabilities. But they can certainly evolve to provide better cognitive testing and decision support tools.

Short-terms goals for the development of better tools should be implemented to enhance the usability features discussed in Section 9.3, as well as the validation processes discussed in Section 9.4.

9.7 Summary

There are several benefits to early detection of dementia. The diagnosis and prognosis can be explained, allowing for planning. It can allow subjects to decide about their wishes to make will, including decisions about future treatments they may wish or not to undergo, such as living wills, participation in clinical trials or consent to autopsy or other research projects.

Periodic cognitive evaluations for elderly people can enhance and elaborate the ability to detect dementia early but are costly, lengthy, and in certain settings even impossible to perform. Computerized methods, if skillfully designed to be useful and usable, can make those large-scale periodical assessments possible.

Several factors may limit the usability of computerized methods. Effects of age, gender, education, and computer experience have to be taken into account, and reference values should be made available. In tests with multiple versions are available in some cases, and their interchangeability must be demonstrated. When adapting a pen-and-paper test, the comparability to the standard must be shown.

As well, there are several confounding factors that have to be controlled for and which can be separated as follows:

9.7.1 Factors Related to the Test Itself

Is the test usable by all subjects? Some obvious limitations are being able to see and sometimes hear, being able to use the keyboard, and so on. Less obvious factors are related to education and literacy. Even if the person can be coached to use the system, the fright of facing an unknown may result in inferior performance.

The validity of the system should be assessed and confirmed, for example, by test–retest evaluations.

9.7.2 Factors Related to the Subject

Normal people fluctuate in their performance depending on distractions and tiredness. Such factors may be even more significant in cognitively impaired individuals. The existence of depression and anxiety may similarly pose an additional challenge and raises the question of whether the performance of depressed persons will be qualitatively different from that of cognitively impaired individuals.

In conventional tests, there is frequently a training effect. Subjects know what to expect in the MMSE and frequently rehearse the answers before entering the examination room. Computer tests can easily bypass the problem by having multiple versions although it must be obvious that they are equivalent to each other.

There is significant ongoing progress in computer technologies, in particular those related to human–computer interaction. Increasing commercial interest in computerized cognitive tools induces proliferation of product developments. These factors imply that current limitations will be diminished and some even eliminated in the coming years, so that more elderly people and health professionals attending to them will be able to enjoy the advantages affordable by computerization.

References

1. Petersen RC, et al. Mild cognitive impairment: clinical characterization and outcome. *Arch Neurol* 1992; 56:303–308.
2. Landauer T K. *The Trouble with Computers*. 1996, MIT Press. ISBN 0262621088.
3. Cooper A. *The Inmates are Running the Asylum*. 2004, McMillan Computer Publishing. ISBN 0672326140.
4. Harvey L. 2004, *Analytic Quality Glossary, Quality Research International*. Available at http://www.qualityresearchinternational.com/glossary.
5. Korczyn AD, Aharonson V. Computerized Methods in the Assessment and Prediction of Dementia. *Current Alzheimer Research* 2007; 4:364–369.
6. Aharonson V, Halperin I, Korczyn AD. Computerized Diagnosis for Mild Cognitive Impairments. Alzheimer's and Dementia 2007; 3:23–7.
7. Aharonson V, Korczyn AD. Human–computer interaction in the administration and analysis of neuropsychological tests. *Comput Methods Programs Biomed* 2004;73:43–53.
8. Aharonson V, Korczyn, AD. *On the Usability of Computerized Cognitive Tests for Dementia Screening*, Prevention of Dementia conference, 2005, Washington, DC.
9. Turing AM, Intelligent machinery, report for National Physical Laboratory, in *Machine Intelligence 7*, B. Meltzer and D. Michie, eds., 1969.

Index

Printed in the United States of America.